THE **COMPLETE GUIDE** TO

ABDOMINAL TRAINING

THE COMPLETE GUIDE TO

Christopher M. Norris

ABDOMINAL TRAINING
3rd edition

A & C Black • London

First published 2009 by
A & C Black Ltd
36 Soho Square, London W1D 3QY
www.acblack.com

Copyright © 2009 Christopher M. Norris

ISBN 978 1 4081 1021 8

Acknowledgements
Cover photography © www.istockphoto.com
Photos © Grant Pritchard, except pp. 1, 2, 3, 9, 128, 143 and 144 Christopher M. Norris
Illustrations © Jeff Edwards

Many thanks to Daniela Levy and Graham Rust for modelling. Thanks also to Peak Fitness in Woking, Surrey, for providing the venue and equipment for the photo shoot.

A & C Black uses paper produced with elemental chlorine-free pulp, harvested from managed sustainable forests.

Typeset in Baskerville by Palimpsest Book Production Limited, Grangemouth, Stirlingshire

Printed and bound in South China by RR Donnelly South China Printing Co

CONTENTS

INTRODUCTION

There are many types of training available today, each with a specific aim. Some aim to reduce weight, others to strengthen muscle, and still others to increase general fitness. Most fashionable abdominal exercise programmes are designed to work the mid-section hard and make the muscles 'hurt', in the belief that this will 'flatten the tummy' or 'trim the waist'. They are often based on long-held traditions, and use terms such as 'going for the burn' and 'pumping up'. Unfortunately, they are not suitable for those of poor or even average fitness levels, firstly because they are too demanding, and secondly because they place excessive stress on the lower back.

The abdominal programme described in this book is very different. It does not come from a sporting background, but from physiotherapy exercises designed to rehabilitate the spine following injury. As such, it aims to be both safe and effective, and to develop trunk fitness which is relevant to everyday life rather than just to sport. Exercise that works in this way is termed 'functional' and this word pervades much of the material in this book. The aim is not to destroy exercise enjoyment, but simply to make it safer and more effective.

– Christopher M. Norris

HOW THE SPINE WORKS

Overview of the spinal column

The human backbone, or spinal column, is made up of 33 individual bones. Each bone is called a *vertebra* (*see* fig. 1.1) and the vertebrae are formed into five groups depending on their location and to a lesser degree their function. In the neck the bones, called *cervical vertebrae*, are delicate but highly mobile, enabling you to turn your head fully. Each vertebra is numbered using a code which indicates its group and position. Cervical vertebrae numbers begin with 'C', thoracic 'T', lumbar 'L' and sacral 'S'. So, for example, the second cervical vertebra counting down from the head is C2, and the fourth is C4. The last lumber vertebra is L5 (rather than L1) because the numbering system begins at the head each time.

Keypoint

Vertebrae are numbered from the head down, with C1 just below the head and C7 between the shoulders.

Fig. 1.1 A vertebra

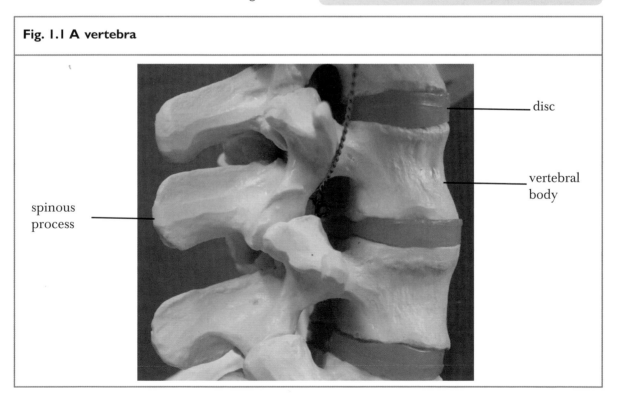

disc

vertebral body

spinous process

The cervical region is subdivided into two functional parts. The upper portion directly below the head is called the *sub-occipital region* (the occiput being the lower back portion of the skull). The C1 and C2 bones make up this region and these two bones are intimately involved in skull movements, especially nodding actions. The lower portion of the neck is called the *lower cervical region* and takes in the bones C3 to C7. This region is more involved with twisting (rotation) and side bending (lateral flexion) actions.

In the chest region the bones are called 'thoracic vertebrae' and these bones connect to the ribs. There are two joints linking the thoracic vertebrae to the ribs: the costovertebral (CV) joint between the vertebral body and the rib, and the costotransverse (CT) joint between the transverse process at the side of the vertebra and the rib angle, where the rib curves to form the drum of the chest (*see* fig. 1.2).

When looking at someone's back, the spinous processes are in the middle, forming a straight column of bumps. The CV joint is about two finger breadths to the side, lying in the furrow of the back. The CT joint is about three finger breadths to the side, covered by the large erector spinae muscles.

Keypoint

In the thoracic spine, the spinous process is in the centre of the back, the costovertebral joint slightly out to the side, and the costotransverse joint further out still.

Fig. 1.2 Joint ribs to thoracic spine

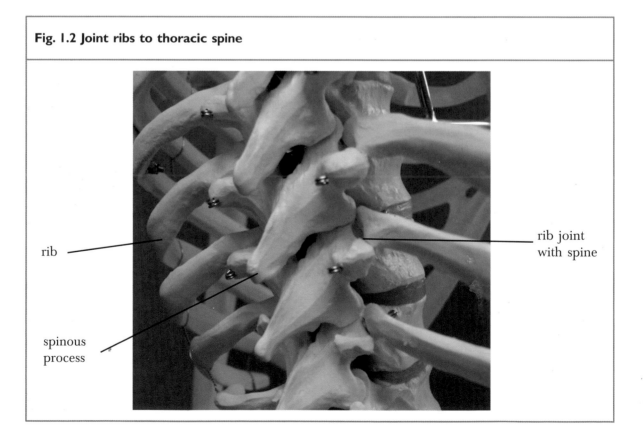

rib

rib joint with spine

spinous process

In the lower spine the spinal bones are called *lumbar vertebrae*. These are large, strong bones covered with powerful muscles. They do not attach to the ribs but their movements are intimately linked to those of the pelvis. The upper portion of the lumbar spine, L1 and L2 move with the thoracic spine, especially during shoulder blade and ribcage movements. The lower lumbar vertebrae, L3/4/5, move closely with the pelvis so that this combined region is often referred to as the lumbo-pelvis.

Below the lumbar vertebrae are the remnants of our tail. The *sacrum* is a triangular-shaped bone which attaches at the sides to the pelvis, while the *coccyx* (*see* fig. 1.3) forms a thin, pointed tip to the end of the spine. Both of these regions are important in terms of injury, especially during pregnancy and childbirth. The joint between the sacrum and the pelvis (sacroiliac joint) is filled with fibrous material and normally gives little movement (*see* fig. 1.4). During childbirth, however, the fibrous material softens and the joint moves to allow the pelvis to expand to facilitate childbirth. This motion can inflame the joint and lead to changes in its alignment. The coccyx again becomes more mobile in this period and can give problems. In addition, in the lean individual, the coccyx is easily damaged by sitting or falling backwards directly onto a hard floor.

Keypoint

The sacroiliac joint joins the sacrum to the pelvis. It is often painful during pregnancy and following childbirth.

Fig. 1.3 A coccyx

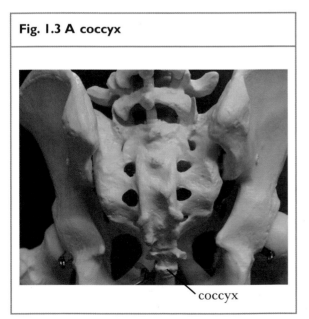

coccyx

Fig. 1.4 Sacrociliac joint

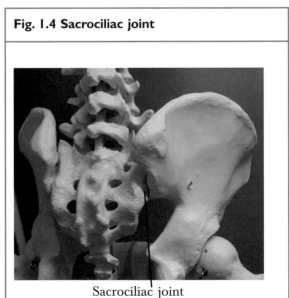

Sacrociliac joint

Spinal curves

Although the spinal vertebrae stand one on top of each other, the column they make is not straight. Instead, the spine forms an 'S' curve. There are two inward curves in the lower back and neck, while the thoracic spine curves gently outwards. These curves are not present at birth but begin to develop in early childhood.

In the early years of life, a baby's spine is rounded, and we call this rounded shape the primary spinal curve (*see* fig. 1.6a). As the baby starts to lie on its front and lift its head up, the neck curve starts to form (*see* fig. 1.6b). It is not until a baby stands up that the curve in the lower back is formed (*see* fig. 1.6c). Because the neck and lower back curves form later, they are called secondary spinal curves.

Fig. 1.6 (a) Primary spinal curve; (b) secondary curve in neck; (c) secondary curve in lower back

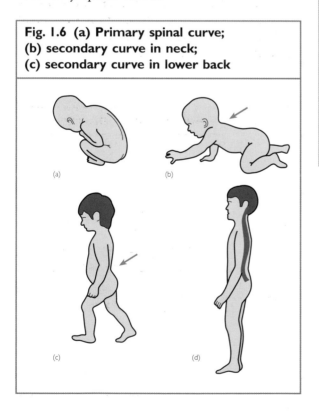

Fig. 1.5 The spinal column

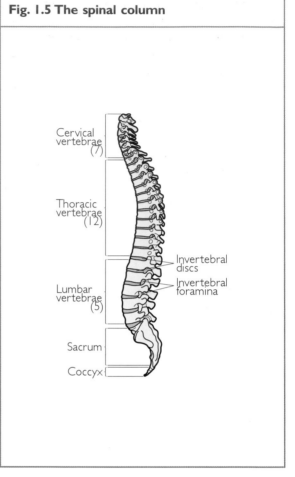

If the spine was completely straight, when we run or jump a large amount of shock would be transmitted up to the head. The function of the spinal curves is to enable the spine to act in a spring-like fashion, absorbing some of the shock of movement and making actions more agile.

When the spinal curves are altered, stress can be placed on the spine. This can occur through alterations in posture and the way we work. Long periods spent sitting at desks and driving a car will change the important curve in the lumbar region and this can be one source of low back pain.

Keypoint

Maintaining a correct curve in the lower back is important to overall spinal health.

Another way that spinal curves can change is through exercise. Training one side of the body excessively can lead to an alteration in muscle balance (one muscle being stronger or tighter than another), pulling the spine out of alignment. This is why a balanced exercise programme is so important. The good news, however, is that the spinal curves can often be helped using specific exercises (exercise therapy) – although this can take some time.

The spinal segment

Each pair of spinal bones together forms a single unit called a 'spinal segment' (*see* fig. 1.7). The two bones are separated by a spongy disc attached to the flat part of the bone. At the back of the vertebra the bone is extended to form two small joints called *facets*. From above, it can

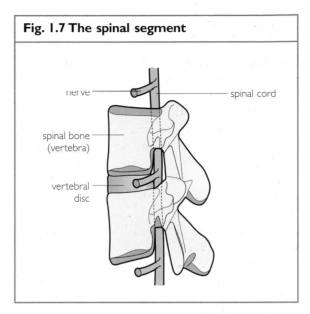

Fig. 1.7 The spinal segment

nerve

spinal cord

spinal bone (vertebra)

vertebral disc

be seen that the back of the spinal bone forms a hollow arch through which runs the spinal cord carrying messages from the brain to the legs and arms (*see* fig. 1.8).

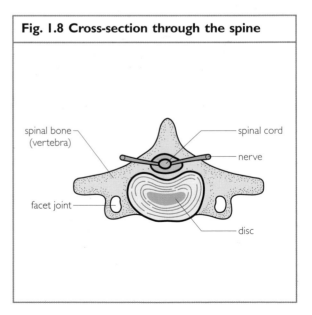

Fig. 1.8 Cross-section through the spine

spinal bone (vertebra)

spinal cord

nerve

facet joint

disc

5

Gym users tend to talk about whole spine movements, bending and straightening, often not realising that segments of the spine can move relative to each other. Instructors should look at specific segments of motion, for example, during an overhead shoulder exercise the thoracic spine may be flattening while the lumbar spine may be curving excessively. Therapists look in even closer detail at the individual spinal segments; they are interested in the motion between L5/L4 relative to that of L4/L3, for example. Motion of an individual spinal segment can be important because stiffness in one segment following injury may cause a neighbouring segment to move excessively (compensatory hypermobility), causing pain. The answer, here, is to make the stiff segment move more so that the lax segment can move less. A physiotherapist will often use joint manipulation to release a stiff spinal segment and then exercise therapy to re-educate the muscles supporting the lax segment.

Keypoint

Look closer at spinal movements. Notice the movement of (i) the whole spine; (ii) regions of the spine relative to each other; (iii) individual spinal segments.

Spinal ligaments

The spine has numerous ligaments but they broadly fall into two categories. There are those running the length of the spine such as the *supraspinous ligament*, those running over the top of the spinous processes, and the *interspinous ligament*, running between the spinous processes. Then there are ligaments associated

with individual joints, such as the *ligamentum flavum* which attaches to the facet joint (*see* fig. 1.9).

Bending forwards will stretch the ligaments behind the spine but relax those in front. Bending backwards will reverse the situation, stretching the front ligaments but relaxing those covering the back of the spine. Movement of an individual spinal segment will stress the ligaments close to that segment and deep beneath the surface of the body.

If you perform an exercise which persistently overstretches a ligament, the ligament will become sore and inflamed. This may take time to develop so you may not feel pain at the time, but you frequently have backache the next day. If this is the case, change your exercise programme.

If a bent position of the spine is held regularly, perhaps as part of your job, overstretched ligaments will lengthen and those which are relaxed will shorten markedly. This is what happens with poor posture. If you are the sort of person who spends most of their day slumped in

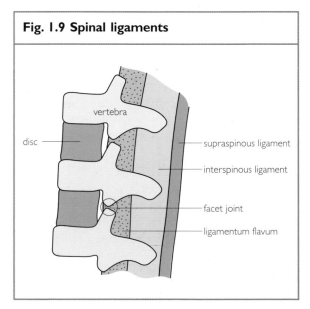

Fig. 1.9 Spinal ligaments

vertebra

disc

supraspinous ligament

interspinous ligament

facet joint

ligamentum flavum

a chair, your spinal ligaments will alter, making it harder for you to hold your spine in a correct alignment when you stand up. To correct this, you must practise exercises to correct your spinal alignment and try to correct your general posture throughout the day.

> ## Keypoint
>
> Repeated bending movements overstretch the spine and can damage it. Cut down on your bending!

Nerves

The spinal cord consists of thousands of tiny nerve fibres bunched together much like a telephone cable. In the same way as the telephone line, the nerves carry electrical messages. When you want to move your leg, for example, an electrical message is sent from the brain. It travels down a nerve contained in your spinal cord to the muscles in your leg, commanding them to move. This is called a *motor function.*

A similar message can move in the opposite direction. If you touch a hot object, an electrical message is sent from your hand up a nerve in your arm through the spinal cord, to the area of brain responsible for feeling, a process called *sensory function.*

At any time, thousands of electrical impulses are travelling up and down the nerves in your body. If something blocks these impulses, the electrical messages change, and both movement (motor function) and feeling (sensory function) can be affected. This is what happens when you trap a nerve. The nerve becomes compressed, a little like stepping on a hose pipe. When this happens the impulses for movement and feeling can become blocked; you get tingling sensations and numbness, and your muscles may twitch or become weak. These sensations can be felt wherever the nerve travels. Often with the lower back, the feelings travel into the buttock and leg and then right down to the foot, a process called *referred pain.*

> ## Keypoint
>
> Pain or 'strange feelings' in your leg could be caused by an injury to your back – a process called referred pain.

The major nerves are covered by a sheath (*see* below) which insulates them in a similar way to that of an electrical cable. Nerve sheaths slide and are stretched during movement. If an injury causes swelling around a nerve, the sheath may tighten both blocking free movement and causing pain or tingling as it is stretched.

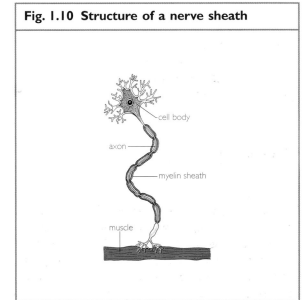

Fig. 1.10 Structure of a nerve sheath

cell body

axon

myelin sheath

muscle

This process, called *adverse neural tension* requires specific stretching exercises targeted at the nerves rather than just the muscles. For details of these stretches see *The Complete Guide to Stretching* by Christopher Norris, published by A&C Black (2007).

Disc structure, function and injury

The disc is the structure which separates the bodies of the two adjacent spinal bones. It acts like a shock absorber, preventing the spine from being shaken or jarred when we walk and run. Each disc has a hard outer casing which contains a softer spongy gel called the 'disc nucleus' (*see* fig. 1.11). Importantly, this gel has no direct blood supply, but instead relies on movement for its health. As the spine moves, fluids are pressed into the disc nucleus and waste products are squeezed out, keeping the disc healthy. As we get older the disc gel begins to dry up and becomes more brittle; the spine gets stiffer, so you are no longer able to turn the cartwheels of your youth when you retire! However,

through regular exercise, the disc stays springy for longer.

If we were to look at the discs of someone who is 30 years old but inactive, and compare them to someone who is 40 but fit, the two discs would probably be exactly the same. The discs of the fitter person have stayed younger because they have been fed through regular movement.

Keypoint

The disc needs regular movement to stay healthy.

Throughout the day, bodyweight compresses the disc and slowly presses water out of it. This compression causes the disc to shrink slightly and reduce its height. Although this is slight, because is occurs throughout the lower spine, the overall effect is a loss of about 1 cm in body height between the morning and evening. Exercises which involve compression either through weight bearing (weight training) or impact (running) also cause the spinal disc to shrink. The loads taken by the spine are magnified through a process of leverage, so a moderate squat exercise can cause compression forces on the L3 and L4 discs of 6–10 times bodyweight. Research has shown that a simple 25-minute weight training session can compress the spine by 5 mm, and a 6 km run by 3 mm. Constant loading with an overhead weight (heavy bodybuilding poundages) can shrink the spine by more than 10 mm. These changes in the lumbar discs make lumbar compression exercises unsuitable for those who have had recent spine problems such as slipped (prolapsed) discs.

As we move the spine, the spinal bones tip forwards and backwards and, as they do so,

---

Fig. 1.11 The structure of the spinal disc

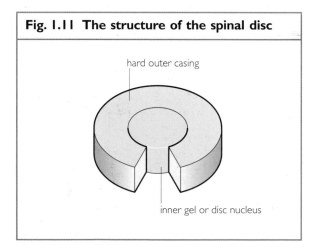

hard outer casing

inner gel or disc nucleus

they press the discs out of shape. When this happens, the gel in the disc is squeezed and its pressure increases. Because we bend forwards much more often than we bend backwards, the gel in the disc starts to move backwards towards the delicate nerves of the spine. When this happens we begin to get pain. Initially this is a dull ache which occurs only occasionally. If we continue to do too much bending, however, we will begin to feel the pain more regularly and it will be more intense as the disc gradually becomes further damaged. Eventually, after many years of repeated bending, the gel in the centre of the disc can burst out and press on to one of the delicate nerves. When this happens it is termed a 'slipped' or more accurately prolapsed disc, a particularly painful condition.

It is important to remember that it is *repeated* bending – stressing the disc over and over again – which is the real villain here. More people suffer from back pain brought on by bending the spine, through slumping in a poor chair or stooping when they work, than from lifting a heavy weight.

Keypoint

Repeated bending squeezes the discs. Over many years damage accumulates and the discs can suddenly burst. This is a slipped or prolapsed disc.

As we will see later, abdominal muscle training has a key role to play in supporting the discs and taking much of the compression forces. Training these muscles is vital after any form of back pain, but the training must be built up gradually; too much, too soon can cause re-injury.

The importance of spinal facet joints

The *facets* are two small joints at the back of the vertebrae (*see* fig. 1.12). Their name comes from the fact that they have flat faces, and the direction in which these are orientated dictates which movements are available in the various spinal regions. In the cervical region the facets are quite round and they face upwards. The thoracic facets are more or less triangular and face backwards. The lumbar facets face upwards and inwards and are larger and stronger than the others. The direction of the facet joints means that very little rotation actually occurs in the lumbar region, rather it occurs mostly in the thoracic spine.

The facet joints are similar in construction to other joints in the body in that they are contained within a tough leathery bag called a *capsule*. As we bend forwards, the facet joint opens up, and as we bend back the joint closes. Twisting the spine results in the surfaces of the facet joint sliding over each other (*see* fig. 1.13).

Because these joints are so small, rapid

Fig. 1.12 The facet joints

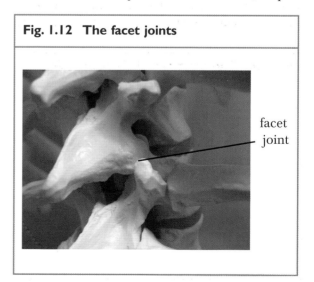

facet joint

Fig. 1.13 Spinal joint movement: (a) bending opens the spinal joints; (b) reaching up closes the spinal joints; (c) twisting causes the spinal joints to slide over each other

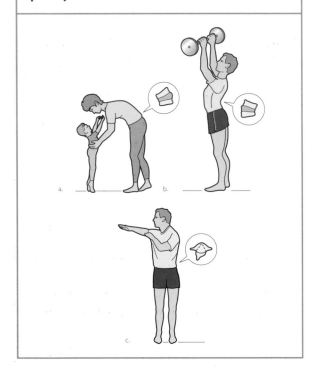

movements can cause them to move too far and so damage them. Bending forwards repeatedly when practising stretching exercises, for example, can overstretch the leathery capsule of the facet joints, leaving the spine looser than it should be and therefore susceptible to injury. Bending backwards suddenly, as can be seen in some weight training exercises, closes the facet joints rapidly with a sudden 'jolt'.

Keypoint

Rapid movements can jolt the small facet joints at the back of the spine over and over again causing pain and swelling.

Over time this can cause premature wearing of these delicate joints.

Range of movement

The total extent of movement which is possible at any joint is called its *range of movement*. Normally, in everyday living, we operate with our joints moving in the middle of this range. This is really the safest part, because the joint is in no danger of being overstretched and the muscles feel comfortable.

With each movement, damage can only occur if the joint is pressed as far as it can go. We call this end point of movement the 'end range'. When we are exercising, if we repeatedly push our joints to the end range we can damage them. A safer method is to practise exercises for which the great majority of movements are in the middle of the movement range. In this way there is a good margin of safety (*see* fig. 1.14).

Keypoint

Exercises which use the middle part of a joint's movement are safer than those which take the joint to the end point of its movement repeatedly.

Lumbar and pelvic movements

Excessive movement in the lumbar spine can occur without us noticing it. If a person bends forwards to touch their toes or backwards to look at the ceiling, the movement is obvious. But another way the lumbar spine can move is more subtle.

The pelvis is connected directly to the

Fig. 1.14 Range of movement

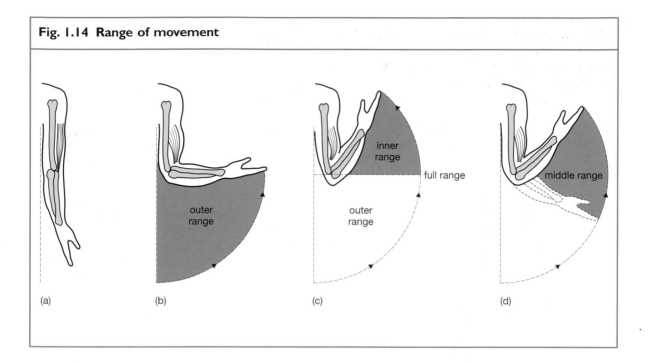

(a)　(b) outer range　(c) inner range / full range / outer range　(d) middle range

Fig. 1.15 Pelvic movement: (a) normal – lower back neutral; (b) forward tilting – lower back hollow; (c) backward tilting – lower back flattens

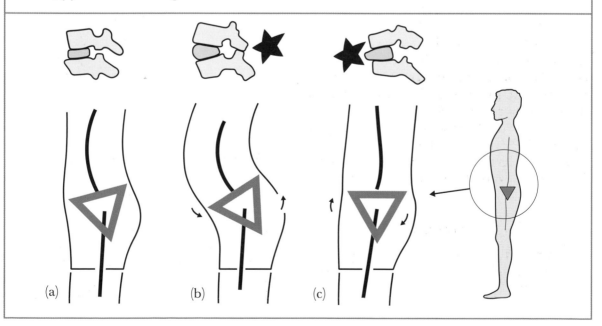

(a)　(b)　(c)

lumbar spine (*see* fig. 1.15) and in turn balances rather like a seesaw on the hip joints. Because it is balanced, the pelvis can tilt forwards and backwards. As it tilts, the pelvis pulls the spine with it. If the pelvis tips down the arch in the lumbar spine increases in a way equivalent to moving the spine backwards into 'extension'. When the pelvis tilts up the lumbar curve is flattened, and the movement in the lumbar spine is equivalent to 'flexion', or forward bending.

If the movement of the pelvis is excessive, the spine in turn is pulled to its end range, stressing the spinal tissues. Note that it is only the lumbar spine which is moving. The rest of the spine remains largely unchanged, so the person is still standing upright.

The ratio between movement of the lumbar

Keypoint

Movement of the pelvis directly affects the lumbar spine.

spine on the pelvis, and movement of the pelvis on the hip joints is important, and this combined motion of both body segments is called the lumbo-pelvic rhythm. When you bend forwards to reach down to a desk from standing, for example, you have a choice. Firstly you could lock your pelvis and bend only from the spine (*see* fig. 1.6a), secondly you could keep your spine stiff and move from your hip alone, or thirdly you could combine the two movements and move from both your hips and spine (*see* fig. 1.6b). The third motion is actually the one which places less stress on the body. By

Fig. 1.16 You could lock your pelvis and bend only from the spine (a), you could keep your spine stiff and move from your hip alone, or you could combine the two movements and move from both your hips and spine (b).

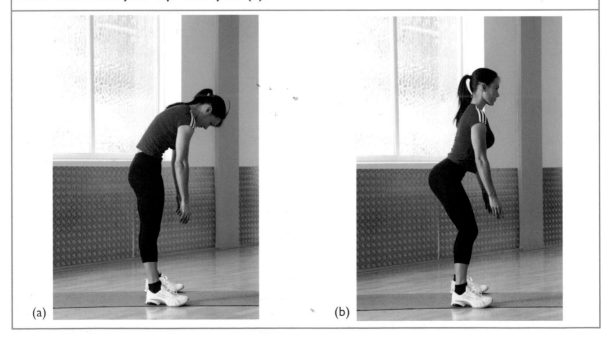

(a) (b)

moving the pelvis on the hips, the requirement for spine bending (lumbar flexion) is reduced and so the lumbar discs are protected. If, however, you keep your spine completely rigid, the lumbar muscles are overworked and can go into spasm causing muscle pain. By allowing the spine to bend and then straighten, the muscles contract and then relax – a more healthy thing to do. Ideally, you should use twice as much pelvic movement as lumbar movement in everyday activities (a lumbo-pelvic ratio of 1:2). Commonly however, people often forget to move from their pelvis and so the lumbar spine does most of the work, giving a lumbo-pelvic ratio of 3:1, with the pelvis moving only when the lumbar spine has moved to its end range.

Keypoint

When bending forwards, the ratio of lumbar movement (flexion) to pelvic movement (anterior tilt) is called the lumbo-pelvic rhythm. Ideally this should be 1:2 when bending for objects at table height.

The neutral position of the lumbar spine

We have seen that, as we move the spine, the alignment of the spinal bones and tissues changes. For example, as we flex forwards, the facet joints open and the tissues on the back of the spine stretch while those on the front relax. At the same time the pressure within the spinal discs increases. This combination of pressure and stretch, if repeated over and over again, can damage the spinal tissues.

If, however, we align the spinal tissues so the spine is upright and the lumbar region is comfortably curved, the spinal tissues are now at their normal length and the pressure within the discs is lowered. We call this normal alignment of the spine the *neutral position*. This is one of the safest postures for the spine, so all the foundation movements that we use begin with the spine in its neutral position.

To find your own neutral position, stand with your back to a wall. Your buttocks and shoulders should touch the wall. Place the flat of your hand between the wall and the small of your back. Try to tilt your pelvis so you flatten your back and then tilt your pelvis the other way so you increase the hollow in the lower back. Your neutral position (and it is slightly different for each person) is halfway between the flat and hollow positions.

You should just be able to place the flat of your hand between your back and the wall. If you can only place your fingers through, your back is too flat; if your whole hand up to your wrist can pass through, your back is too hollow (*see* page 11).

Keypoint

In the neutral position the spine is correctly aligned and the spinal tissues are held at the right length.

To find the neutral position on a client (*see* fig. 1.17 overleaf) or training partner, have them stand up against a wall with their hands out in front, arms straight (standing press-up position). Stand behind them side on and, with their permission, reach your left forearm around their waist placing it across their waistband. Press your left shoulder against the back of their ribcage (*see* fig. 1.17a) and the flat of your right hand over their sacrum. Their upper body is effectively fixed by their hands on the wall (they must keep their arms straight) and your left shoulder pressing against the back of their

Fig. 1.17 Finding neutral position on a client

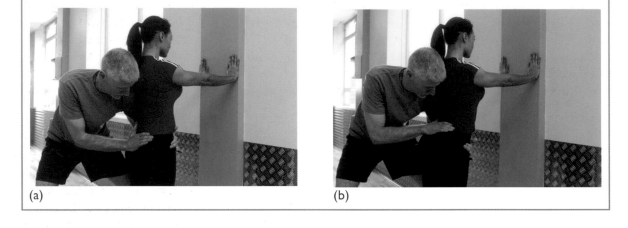

(a)   (b)

ribcage. Your left hand monitors the front of their pelvis and your right the back (sacrum). Using this position you can help them to tilt their pelvis using your hands to guide or 'cue' the movement (*see* fig. 1.17b). Using touch in this fashion to give feedback is called *tactile cueing* and is an effective way of teaching, often cutting down many frustrating hours of practice for a client. Initially, simply tilt the pelvis to encourage full range movement, and then stop in the neutral position.

Keypoint

Use tactile cueing to help a partner find neutral position of the lumbar spine.

Core stability

If we can maintain the neutral position of the spine when we move or lift, for example, we can greatly reduce the stress on the spinal tissues. This is an essential part of the concept of core stability (back stability). In simple terms, core stability literally means holding the centre

part of the body firm so that the limbs (arms and legs) will have a stable base upon which to move. The concept of holding one part firm so that another part can move effectively is not new, of course, and is seen in all sorts of common daily activities. When we drive a car, for example, we put our foot on the accelerator and expect the car to go forward. For this to happen, the tyre must grip on the road surface and the road must stay firm or 'stable'. If the tyre grips on ice instead, the wheel simply spins and forward movement of the car cannot occur.

Interacting components of stability

The core of the body is the part between the pelvis and the ribcage, and this relies on muscle to hold it firm. Core stability results from the interplay between three body components (*see* fig. 1.18). The first is the shape of the bones and joints. This is called the *passive* component because it is moved by muscles or forces *outside* the body, such as heavy weight, but is not able to move by itself. If the passive system breaks down, the body core will loose stability. A broken bone, or dislocated joint, for example, will leave the body virtually unable to move because the body part is insecure. No matter how much we pull or push on it, the pain and instability will stop us moving effectively. The body quite rightly recognises that this will damage us and forces us to rest.

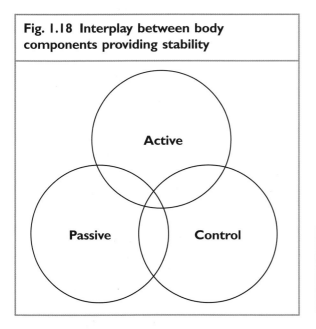

Fig. 1.18 Interplay between body components providing stability

The next component which contributes to core stability is the *active* system. This is made up of the muscles which pull on the bones and joints either to hold them firm or to move them. In order to do this effectively, the muscles must be sufficiently strong. Using an example of a broken bone, if we place the limb in a plaster cast the bone will heal: the *passive* system (bone) therefore becomes more solid or stable. However, when we remove the plaster cast all the muscles will have wasted and we are both too weak to move the limb very far, and too weak to hold it firm (stable). This is why after a fracture the

leg often 'gives way' when we twist or turn suddenly. The passive stability (bone) is fine, but the active stability (muscle) is weak.

When the muscles become strong, we cannot use them all the time because they will get tired, and we do not want tense muscles continually. The ideal situation is to be able to turn the muscles on and off so that we can use them to stabilise the body when we need them to and allow them to rest when we don't. Economy of movement is the key here, and this is the job of the third stability component, *control*. This system works by the brain and spinal cord monitoring tiny sensors in the joints and muscles of the body. These sensors give us information about body position, movement, and stress and strain which is imposed on the body through everyday activities. When a joint or body part is put under strain, the sensors will detect this and send a message to the muscles to tighten and hold that part of the body firm – or 'stabilise' it – to resist the forces stressing it.

Keypoint

Core stability relies on passive (bone and ligament) active (muscle) and control (coordination) systems.

This process of force detection and muscle reaction is the job of the control system. In some people this is very good and runs extremely smoothly. In a ballet dancer, for example, the muscles may be small and lean, but because the body control is very good the dancer can use just the right amount of muscle force to hold the body stable and control each action with great precision. After a knee injury, a rugby player may still have much bigger muscles than the ballet dancer, but through pain the body control has been lost. The muscles shake and quiver as the knee is moved and the actions are ungainly and poorly controlled.

In the case of the lumbar spine, which is clearly in the centre of the body, the stability provided by the active, passive and control systems is the *core* of the body. In this case the active system is that of the abdominal and lumbar muscles (*see* pages 18–20), while the passive system consists of the spinal bones, discs and ligaments. The control system integrating these two comes from nervous impulses in both the spine and brain. The muscles of the active sub-system can be divided into the surface (superficial) muscles of the rectus abdominis and the external obliques which primarily move the core region, and the deeper muscles, transversus abdominis and internal obliques which mainly *prevent excessive movement* of the body core and 'stabilise' it.

> ### Keypoint
>
> It is the muscle's function not just to *create* movement, but to *protect* the body against excessive motion created from external forces acting upon it.

Thus, for effective core stability, a subtle interplay between the three stability systems is required. The bones and joints must move freely, the muscles must be strong and supple, and the body control must be well coordinated. Failure of any one of these systems will reduce core stability. Importantly, however, if this does occur, correctly applied exercise can often build up the other two stability components to compensate. Take arthritis as an example; in this condition there is wear and tear of the joints. This can often leave the joint less stable with a tendency to give way. In this situation, a physiotherapist can give a patient special exercises to strengthen the muscles which support the joint and improve the body control by using skilled movements. The *active* and *control*

components of stability are therefore built up to compensate for the *passive* system which is worn. Although the bones cannot be changed, the patient enjoys virtually full, pain-free actions because the body has compensated for the damaged joints and bones.

Local and global muscles

We have two sets of muscles contributing to core stability (*see* page 35). Some are close to the central core of the body and are called *local* muscles. Others are quite far away from the central core and are called *global* muscles. The local muscles, close to the spine and pelvis, act to move the spine subtly and adjust it with fine movements to keep the posture correct and make sure the body alignment is optimal. The global muscles, on the other hand, do not make fine adjustments of spinal position, but instead take some of the strain on the body before this strain can damage the spine. When lifting, for example, the large leg muscles (global) can be used to provide the power for the lift while the deep muscle corset (local) can maintain the neutral position of the lower spine.

Often, after a bout of back pain, the local muscles are turned off and quickly waste (become lax). When we move, we lose subtle movements of the spine and rely instead on our large global muscles. Our movements become clumsy and poorly coordinated, and the muscles often become tight, tense and painful. Our back feels stiff after a bout of gardening, for example, and the muscles feel tight and cord-like. Instead of using the subtle local musculature of the body core, we have used the strong global muscles. They are too powerful for this task, however, and quickly go into spasm, giving pain. If we make the mistake of trying to strengthen the back in a gym using heavy weight training techniques, these already firm global muscles can be built up even further without the subtle local muscles being worked, so we end up with an imbalance between the two sets of muscles resulting in further pain.

The gentle foundation movements given in this book are designed to restore muscle balance and work to improve core stability, because they target the local muscles. Once these have been performed and core stability has been improved, the exercises gradually bring in the global muscles to build complete 'spinal fitness'.

Keypoint

Lax muscles can give pain by allowing parts of the body to move excessively, stressing joints. *Tight* muscles can be painful simply through spasm. Both sets of muscles should be addressed during a corrective exercise programme.

Summary

- The spine is divided into regions: *cervical* (neck), *thoracic* (ribcage), *lumbar* (lower back), *sacrum* and *coccyx* (tailbone).
- The lower spine and pelvis together form the lumbo-pelvis.
- The spine forms an 'S' curve, making it naturally springy.
- Bending and straightening the spine stretches and relaxes the spinal ligaments.
- Nerves transmit electrical messages for movement and feeling.
- If a nerve is trapped, movement and feeling can alter, giving weakness, pain or tingling.
- Referred pain is pain travelling to another part of the body from the original area of injury.
- The spinal disc contains a gel and acts as a shock-absorber.
- Safe movement keeps the spinal discs healthy, but poor movement allows stress to build in the discs over many years.
- Mid-range is the centre part of the total extent of movement possible at a joint.
- In its neutral position, the spine is correctly aligned and the spinal tissues are at their normal length.
- Back stability depends on the interaction between the *passive* (bones), *active* (muscle) and *control* (coordination) components of the body.
- Muscles *local* to the spine control the subtle position of the spinal bones. Muscles some distance away from the spine (*global*) help to minimise forces before they reach the spine.

THE TRUNK MUSCLES

2

We need to become familiar with all of the muscles affecting the lower trunk – the area between the ribcage and the pelvic bones. At the front and sides of the trunk are the four principal *abdominal muscles*, at the back the *spinal muscles* and, at the base of the trunk, and actually within the pelvic bones themselves, the *pelvic floor muscles*. We are also concerned with the hip muscles because, as we have seen, hip, pelvic, and lumbar motion is intimately linked.

In the centre of the abdomen is the *rectus abdominis* (*see* fig. 2.1a). This muscle runs from the lower ribs to the pubic region, forming a narrow strap. It tapers down from about 15 cm (6 inches) wide at the top to 8 cm (3 inches) wide at the bottom. The muscle has three fibrous bands across it at the level of the tummy button, and above and below this point. The rectus muscle on each side of the body is contained within a sheath; the two sheaths merge in the centre line of the body via a strong fibrous band called the *linea alba*. This region

---

Fig. 2.1 The abdominal and hip flexor muscles

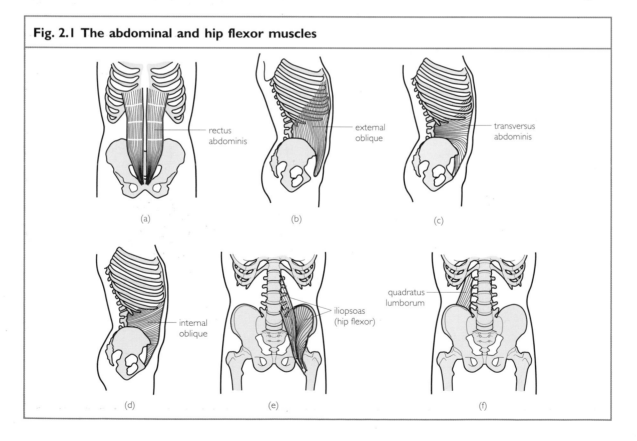

rectus abdominis

external oblique

transversus abdominis

(a)　　　　(b)　　　　(c)

internal oblique

iliopsoas (hip flexor)

quadratus lumborum

(d)　　　　(e)　　　　(f)

splits during pregnancy to allow for the bulk of the developing child (*see* chapter 14).

At the side of the abdomen there are two diagonal muscles, the internal oblique (*see* fig. 2.1d) and the external oblique (*see* fig. 2.1b). The internal oblique attaches to the front of the pelvic bone and a strong ligament in this region. From here it travels up and across to the lower ribs and into the sheath covering the rectus muscle. The external oblique has a similar position, but lies at an angle to the internal oblique. The external oblique begins from the lower eight ribs and travels to the sheath covering the rectus muscle and to the strong pelvic ligaments. The fibres in the centre of the muscle are travelling diagonally, but those right on the edge are travelling vertically and will assist the rectus muscle in its action.

Underneath the oblique abdominals lies the

transversus abdominis (*see* fig. 2.1c). This attaches from the pelvic bones and tissue covering the spinal muscles and travels horizontally forwards to merge with the sheath covering the rectus muscle.

Fig. 2.2 shows a cross-section of the trunk. In the centre you can see the rectus muscle surrounded by connective tissue called the rectus sheath. This sheath from the two neighbouring muscles joins in the centre to form the linea alba. At the side of the trunk you can see the three distinct layers of muscles, from the

---

Fig. 2.2 A cross-section of the trunk

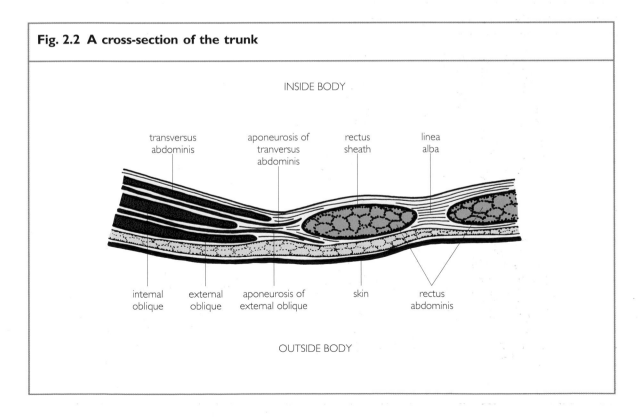

---

inside out transversus, internal oblique and external oblique.

At the side and back of the trunk, the *quadratus lumborum* muscle is also important (*see* fig. 2.1f). It is positioned between the pelvis and ribcage, and has an inner and outer portion. The inner portion is attached directly to the spine, so is important for stability. The outer portion has a tendency to get tight and painful during backpain.

There are several hip muscles, but the most important in relation to abdominal training is the *iliopsoas* (*see* fig. 2.1e). This is, in fact, two muscles (the psoas and iliacus) attached to a single point on the hip. The psoas muscle attaches to various parts of the lumbar spine including the vertebra itself and the spinal disc – hence its importance to the spine. The iliacus muscle attaches from the inner surface of the pelvis and has no direct effect on the spine. Both muscles travel forwards to the inner/upper part of the thigh bone (femur). The iliopsoas works to lift the thigh upwards (hip flexion) or the trunk downwards towards the thigh when this bone is fixed (sit-up action). The muscle also causes compression of the spine when it is worked hard in, for example, a straight leg lifting action lying on the back.

Keypoint

The iliopsoas muscle of the hip affects the spine by (i) lifting the trunk in a sit-up action; and (ii) causing lumbar compression forces during a straight leg lifting motion.

When we are performing abdominal exercises to enhance core stability we must also be aware of the pelvic floor muscles (*see* fig. 14.2, page 174). These attach to the inside of the pelvis and form a sort of sling running from the tailbone (coccyx), at the back, to the pubic bone (crotch) at the front. The muscles from each side of the body join in the middle, and the front and back passages (vagina, urethra and anus) are formed within the pelvic floor muscles. These openings are controlled by rings of muscle called *sphincters* which lie in the pelvic floor. The pelvic floor muscles are important for both men and women. They are essential for core stability following back pain and may be damaged in women during pregnancy and in men following prostate surgery (*see* chapter 14).

Keypoint

The pelvic floor muscles are important in both men and women.

All these muscles work together and so, in any action involving the abdomen, most of the muscles will be active to a certain extent. In a sit-up action, the iliopsoas works and the upper portion of the rectus is emphasised. In pelvic tilting the lower portion of the rectus and the outer fibres of the external oblique are used. Twisting actions involve the oblique abdominals, while the transversus acting with the obliques pulls the tummy in tight. This muscle is used in coughing and sneezing as well. Together with the obliques, the outer portion of the quadratus is important for side bending actions and also pulls on the lower ribs when breathing deeply. The inner portion is next to the spine and helps to support it in actions which tend to pull you sideways. The quadratus is therefore important to core stability when carrying an object in one hand – for example, a shopping basket or case. After pregnancy (*see* chapter 14), following certain types of lower back pain, after some types of surgery and in very obese individuals, the pelvic floor muscles reduce their tone and people can sometimes lose control of the sphincters and dribble urine. For this reason, regaining control of the pelvic floor is important and can be achieved at the same time as re-educating the deep muscle corset (transversus and internal oblique). As we shall see (on page 174), the pelvic floor muscles are also integral to the creation of pressure which forms the 'abdominal balloon', an important process in developing core stability.

Summary

- The rectus muscle bends the trunk and lifts the tail when lying on the back.
- The obliques twist the spine.
- The transversus pulls the tummy in tight.
- The quadratus lumborum muscle stiffens the spine when a force tries to bend the spine sideways.
- The iliopsoas flexes the hip and compresses the lumbar spine.
- The pelvic floor muscles can be re-educated at the same time as core stability.

How the trunk muscles act for core stability

There are several methods by which the trunk muscles can make the trunk more solid and contribute to core stability.

The abdominal balloon

If we look at the trunk we can imagine it as a cylinder (*see* fig. 2.3). The walls of the cylinder are the oblique abdominal muscles which form the deep muscle corset (transversus,

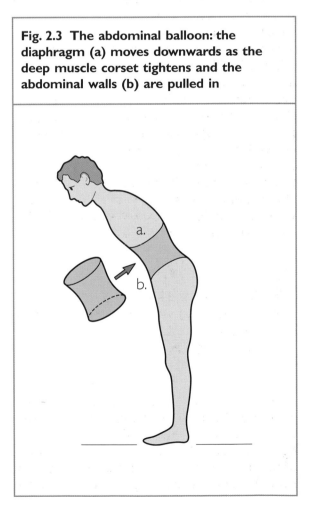

Fig. 2.3 The abdominal balloon: the diaphragm (a) moves downwards as the deep muscle corset tightens and the abdominal walls (b) are pulled in

internal obliques and multifidus). The top of the cylinder is formed by the diaphragm, a sheet of muscle tissue which 'cuts the body in half' and is found beneath the chest and above the tummy. This muscle enables us to breathe, pulling air into the lungs and forcing it out again like a pair of bellows. When we breathe in, the diaphragm goes down to pull air into the lungs. Because it goes down, the top of our 'cylinder' is squashed in, much like pressing on the top of a drinks can, for example. The floor of the cylinder is formed by the pelvic floor muscles, the ones which make us 'hold on' when we are desperate to go to the toilet but can't find the bathroom! When we do this, these muscles are pulled into the body slightly, giving us the feeling that we are pulling in and upwards between the legs.

Keypoint

The abdominal balloon is created by the abdominal muscles, pelvic floor muscles, and diaphragm.

When all three sets of muscles work together, the cylinder is squeezed in every direction: the top is pulling down, the bottom is pulling up, and the walls are squeezing inwards. Contained within the cylinder are the stomach, intestines and body organs and, as the muscles squeeze in, the whole area acts like a giant balloon, providing a solid 'bubble' at the front of the trunk. As we lift a heavy object there is a tendency for the spine to buckle and bend forwards (flex), but the abdominal balloon – positioned at the front of the body – helps to stop this happening.

Heavy lifts or rapid movements of the trunk result in stronger muscle contractions and so the pressure produced by the abdominal balloon is greater. As this pressure is within the abdomen, it is called *Intra Abdominal Pressure*,

or IAP. The larger the IAP, the better a person's core stability, and this is achieved by having deep abdominal muscles which are strong but, more importantly, able to hold the area firm for long periods. This is why holding, or muscle endurance, is important to core stability (*see* page 32).

Interestingly, because all three sets of muscles which form the cylinder have to tighten at the same time, the coordination of this action can break down. One example of this is the incontinence which some young mums suffer. This occurs sometimes when they cough or laugh, because both of these actions increase the IAP. Although the pressure is increasing, the pelvic floor muscles are poorly toned and poorly controlled after pregnancy and so the pressure causes urine (water) to press out of the bladder unrestrained. The answer is to restore the feeling that the muscles between the legs are pulling 'in and up' by using special pelvic floor exercises and also targeting the deep muscle corset (*see* page 174).

Keypoint

Intra Abdominal Pressure (IAP) is the inward squeezing force created as the muscles forming the abdominal balloon tighten.

Back fascia

The second method by which core stability is created involves a sheet of tough elastic material which stretches from the back of the ribcage to the pelvis. The material is called *fascia*, and because this particular piece stretches across the upper back (thoracic spine) and lower back (lumbar spine) it is called the Thoraco-Lumbar Fascia or TLF. As we lift an object and are pulled forwards by its weight, the fascia is stretched. However, several muscles work to pull on the fascia and tighten it, enabling it to resist this force because:

- The transversus muscle and the internal oblique surround the trunk and attach at the back to the fascia. When they tighten they pull the fascia from the sides, similar to the effect of pulling on the side of someone's shirt to flatten it.
- The back muscles (spinal extensors) are two strong vertical columns running up either side of the spine. They are encased in a layer of the fascia, and when they contract they also stretch the fascia and tighten it.
- The buttock muscles (gluteals) and the muscles which pull your arms to your sides (latissimus dorsi) connect to the top and bottom of the fascia. They tighten it by

pulling the TLF upwards and downwards at the same time as the deep abdominal muscles pull it sideways.

The net result of all this muscular activity is to strengthen the spine and help it resist the bending forces which are seen in lifting. They create an effective mechanism, but one which will only be able to function optimally if the muscles are strong and able to pull for a long period of time. In addition, the muscles must work at the right time in a lift. If they pull too soon their force will do no good, and if they pull after the weight has been lifted, the stress will already have been placed on the spine. Again, coordination is important. The muscles must pull at just the right time, with just the right amount of force – and, after a bout of back pain or a long period of inactivity, this mechanism takes training and practice to restore.

Fig. 2.4 The back fascia: (a) latissimus dorsi; (b) gluteals and (c) internal oblique, transverses

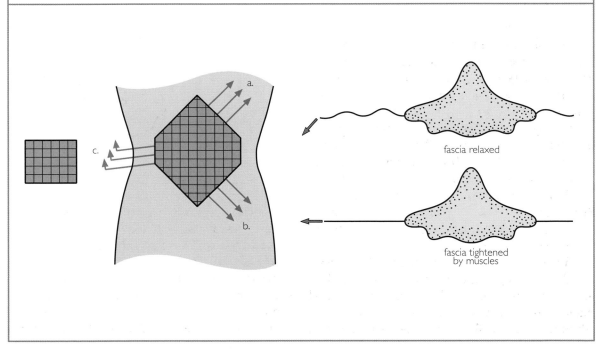

fascia relaxed

fascia tightened by muscles

Fig. 2.5 Cross-section of the trunk

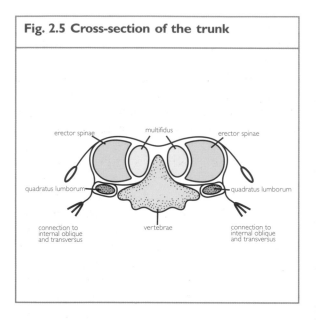

erector spinae · multifidus · erector spinae

quadratus lumborum · quadratus lumborum

connection to internal oblique and transversus · vertebrae · connection to internal oblique and transversus

Keypoint

The deep abdominals, gluteals, erector spinae, and latissimus muscles connect to the thoracolumbar fascia (TLF). By tightening it, these muscles help stabilise the spine.

Back extensor muscles

There are two groups of back extensor muscles which are important to core stability, especially in lifting. The first are local muscles which attach each of the vertebrae covering a single spinal segment. The second are global muscles (*see* page 16) which attach along the whole length of the spine, spanning several spinal segments.

Of the local group, the *multifidus* muscle is particularly important. This not only moves the spinal bones in relation to each other – in other words, it produces a rocking action of one bone against the other in the same way as one brick can move within a column of bricks – but also flattens the lumbar curve without moving the whole spine. Probably the most important feature of this muscle, however, is its ability to stiffen the spine. Because it is positioned between the spinal bones, it acts a little like cement between bricks. A column of bricks stacked on top of each other is very unstable. However, if the bricks are cemented together with mortar, they are very stable, any amount of pressing and pulling will be withstood, and the column will remain standing. The multifidus has a similar function in that it stiffens the spine and helps it to resist bending forces. However, after a back injury or bout of low back pain, it becomes much smaller and weaker and so the spine is more susceptible to further injury. Unfortunately, when the back pain has been resolved, the multifidus does not build itself back up again readily. It needs to be 'reminded' how to work, through the use of special exercises.

Keypoint

The multifidus muscle supports the spine by making it stiffer and better able to resist unwanted bending stresses. The muscle often wastes and weakens after back injury.

The global spinal muscles are the spinal extensors which lie on either side of the spine. These consist of several muscles, the two most important being a central muscle (*longissimus*) which travels close to the spine and a more side-placed muscle (*iliocostalis*) which attaches to the ribs. Together, they are like two powerful columns which support the spine as we bend forwards and move the back from the vertical to a more horizontal position. Although the strength of these muscles is important, their endurance (how long they can hold themselves tight) is actually more significant. This is because if the endurance of the muscles is poor, they will gradually allow the back to slip into an increasingly poor posture after repeated bending activities.

Think of the spine as a fishing rod. Instead of only heavy fish causing the rod to bend enticingly, the rod has weakened so that *any* fish caught on the line looks like a whopper! The result is the same. The rod, or in this case the spine, bends more and more. Therefore the amount of time someone can spend tightening the back muscles and holding them tight is the important factor, especially with intensive activities such as sport or heavy lifting. This is why we target these muscles with a number of exercises, ultimately leading to the spinal extension hold shown on page 157. The way that you lift an object and the function of your spine as a lever during your lifting posture is covered in chapter 4.

against. If not, the force created by the limbs will move the trunk rather than the object intended.

Any of the trunk muscles can be activated by appropriate exercises to move the spine. However, to stabilise the spine it is the muscles deep inside the body, and therefore closer to the spine, which are used. The transversus and the deep back muscles (quadratus lumborum and multifidus) are some of your most important stability muscles, and they are helped by the internal oblique. The rectus muscle, external oblique, and erector spinae (the muscles nearer the surface of the back) are responsible for rapid movements such as sitting up from lying; twisting; or standing up straight again from a bent over position. They are important for spinal health, but not immediately for stability.

Keypoint

The amount of time someone can tighten the back muscles and hold them tight (endurance) is more important than pure strength.

Keypoint

The deep trunk muscles make the spine more stable, holding the spinal bones together. The muscles on the surface are better at causing movement. Both are vital to spinal health.

Selecting which muscles to work

The abdominal muscles can either be used for *movement*, to bend or twist the trunk, for example, or for *stability*. When used for stability, the muscles hold the spine firm, preventing excessive movement. In order to do this, they work to make the trunk into a more solid cylinder. For instance, when we are lifting something or pushing and pulling, the spine has to form a solid base for the arms and legs to push

The hip muscles

The major hip muscle affected during abdominal training is the *hip flexor* (iliopsoas). As we saw in chapter 1, it attaches in two parts. The first part coming from the lumbar spine, the second from the pelvis (*see* fig. 2.1e). Both parts merge to fasten on to the top of the thighbone (femur). The action of this muscle is best illustrated when lying flat on your back. If you lift one leg, the hip flexor has acted to bend the hip. If you sit up from lying flat, keeping your back straight and bending at the hip, the muscle has acted to pull your trunk up.

Because the muscle attaches to each vertebra of the lumbar spine, as it contracts it will pull the lumbar vertebrae together. As this happens, the pressure within the vertebra will increase. This has two effects, one good and one bad. Slight pressure will help to hold the vertebra in place, stabilising them. As pressure increases further, however, the spinal discs can distort causing them to press closer to the nerves in the area, causing pain. This effect is made greater when the spine is not optimally aligned – too bent or too hollow. Minimising (but not obliterating) work of the iliopsoas during abdominal training, and ensuring that the low back is in its neutral position when the iliopsoas is working, is a key feature of good abdominal exercise practice in general, but especially when someone is just starting out.

Keypoint

If the iliopsoas muscle is worked too hard it can pull excessively on the lower spine, dangerously increasing the pressure within the discs.

How muscles cause movement

Muscle consists of many fibres running parallel to each other. If we look through a microscope at these fibres we see that they contain a series of interlocking finger-like projections. When a muscle contracts, the finger-like projections pull together and overlap, shortening the muscle. So, as a muscle contracts it will pull; it cannot push. For example, if you bend your arm the muscles on the inside of the arm pull the forearm towards

the upper arm. The muscles on the outside of the arm cannot push the arm into this position; they must actually relax to allow the movement to occur.

Keypoint

A muscle can only pull; it cannot push.

The more the finger-like projections within the muscle can overlap, the stronger the muscle will be. If the muscle starts from a position where the projections are already overlapped and the muscle is shortened, the force the muscle can produce is very small, because there is little further movement available. If the muscle is overstretched, the finger-like projections can't overlap sufficiently and so, again, the muscle appears weak. For maximum strength gains, the muscle should be contracted from a comfortable lengthened position, not too short (cramped) or overstretched.

The other function of a muscle is to act like a giant elastic band. When stretched, the tissue within the muscle will spring back, and we call this 'recoil' or *elastic strength*. When we look at the abdominal muscles during an exercise, we must consider how each muscle is acting to create a movement, and how it could limit a movement because of its length.

Elastic strength of a muscle is more important for the large leg muscles, such as the hamstrings (back of the thigh) and rectus femoris (front of the thigh). These muscles are thick and stocky in cross section. The elastic strength that they possess comes from recoil of the muscle itself, and the material which surrounds the muscle fibres (the muscle sheath). This surrounding sheath is made from connective tissue. Because the leg muscles are stocky, they have a lot of muscle fibres to string back. This structure is similar for the rectus abdominis muscles at the centre of the trunk; its stocky 'six pack' nature make elastic strength quite important in advanced training during power sports.

The oblique abdominal muscles, which surround the trunk, however, are different in their make-up. They are thin and sheet-like. Although their fibres are thin, they are covered in sheets of connective tissue and when they contract, rather than bulging like the leg or arm muscles, they flatten and the muscle sheet becomes firmer. Their function is better suited to pulling inwards and supporting the body organs (called *visceral compression*), holding the trunk firm when you are pushing, pulling and lifting (stability).

Muscle and movement dysfunction

When muscles don't work correctly, we call them *dysfunctional*. The change in the way that they work will alter body movement in general, and this is therefore termed *movement dysfunction*. Almost always the reverse process is true; movement dysfunction gives rise to muscle changes. Over time, these changes can become almost permanent and there is a change in the muscle structure.

Keypoint

Structure and function are intimately linked. Alteration in the way we move (function) can change muscle make-up (structure). Change in muscle make-up will in turn change the way we move.

Let's look at an example to illustrate the link between structure and function in the body. Imagine that you are playing squash and your opponent strikes the ball hard and it hits you in the side. It hurts, and bruises quite badly. Over the next couple of days there will be both structural and functional changes in your body. The area will swell slightly, and bruise: both changes in structure – one concerning lymph fluid (swelling) the other blood (bruising). Because the area is painful, you tend to lean over towards the injured side (left side flexion in the case of left trunk bruising) to take the stretch off the area and reduce pain. This is a functional change – you are simply choosing to side-flex your trunk. Over time, however, because you have leant over for so long it becomes a habit and we call this a *habitual posture change*. Your body adapts to this change by shortening the muscles on the side to which you lean (left) and lengthening the opposite side muscles (right). The *functional change* of simply leaning over has now become a *structure change* of shortened and lengthened muscle.

To reverse this process we must address both structure and function. Simply telling someone to stand up straight is not sufficient with a long-term postural change. However hard they try, they cannot easily pull against the tight muscle which has changed its structure. A physiotherapist may need to use special techniques (manual therapy) to release the muscle and then rehabilitation exercises to begin postural correction. This is then taken over by a personal trainer who can guide a client through a series of exercises to re-educate body alignment.

Abdominal muscle changes

There are three typical changes that we need to address in the abdominal region. Changes due to weight gain (obesity), pregnancy (chapter 14) and following a surgical operation (chapter 16). The last two we will look at later in the book, so now let's concern ourselves with changes to the abdominal muscles during obesity.

For the actual definition of obesity and its relation to body mass index (BMI) and waist measurement *see* chapter 5.

Normally, the sheet-like abdominal muscles combined with deep sheets of connective tissue (peritoneum) hold the abdominal organs in place. When we stand up, the organs do not fall down; they are supported. As we gain weight, however, the increasing weight of the tissue begins to stretch the abdominal muscles, and the organs move forwards slightly. The force of gravity pulls them downwards, and the combined forward and downward movement of the body organs is called *visceral ptosis*. As the organs move forwards they are moving away from the body gravity line (*see* chapter 4) and so, in effect, getting heavier. This means that, once started, the process can accelerate

quite quickly. The abdominal muscles are stretched and the skin also stretches, often developing stretch marks (striae) as the skin itself is microscopically torn and repaired.

To correct the visceral ptosis, a combined approach is required. The weight of the abdomen must be reduced by diet and the abdominal muscles must be strengthened and shortened. These are both structural changes. To fully correct the visceral ptosis, however, the habitual posture (a functional change) must also be addressed. Abdominal hollowing actions and correct postural alignment must be regularly practised throughout the day, and incorporated into an exercise programme. Activities which emphasise good postural alignment, such as Pilates and yoga, are ideal.

BASIC CONCEPTS OF ABDOMINAL TRAINING

3

Effective muscle strengthening

For a muscle to become stronger, it must be worked harder than it would be in everyday activities. When it is, we say that the muscle has been overloaded. To achieve this degree of muscle work, we must decide on the type of exercise required, and its duration, frequency of use and intensity. These are called the *training variables* (*see* table 3.1), and altering any of them will change the overall work intensity. The total amount of work is often expressed in sets and reps and, together, the description of an exercise using these variables is commonly referred to as *training volume*. For example, heavy weight training is clearly harder than light jogging (exercise type), while slow walking is easier than fast walking (intensity). Performing a trunk curl exercise every hour throughout the day is harder than performing it every other day (frequency), and performing 10 repetitions is easier than 100 repetitions (duration). Performing the trunk curl everyday for 3 sets of 10 repetitions gives a larger training volume than performing it three times each week for 2 sets of 12 repetitions.

When we are trying to strengthen the abdominal muscles, the type of exercise will dictate the type of strength we will build up. There are three major sorts of strength, termed *isometric, concentric* and *eccentric*. Isometric strength occurs when we tense a muscle and hold it tight. It is the type of strength needed to hold a joint still and to stop it moving, so is important to stability. Concentric strength occurs when a muscle is shortening and speeding up a movement. It is the type used when we pick something up, for example. Eccentric strength is exactly the reverse. During eccentric activity, the muscle begins to lengthen and is gradually 'let out'. It is the type of activity used when lowering a weight in a controlled fashion, or when leaning over a desk to put a book down.

The three types of muscle work can be further illustrated when standing up and sitting down in a chair. As we stand up, the thigh muscles are tightening and working concentrically. If we stop ourselves just short of full standing and hold the position, the same muscles work isometrically. As we slowly lower ourselves down again back into the chair, the muscles are working eccentrically. All three

Table 3.1	Training variables
Variable	**Meaning**
Type	Exercise category (weight training, stretching etc.)
Duration	How long exercise lasts
Frequency	How often exercise is practiced (daily, weekly etc)
Intensity	How hard exercise is

types of muscle work are important to the abdominals, and so all three are used in this programme.

The intensity (how hard), duration (how long) and frequency (how often) of exercises used in an abdominal training programme is also important: too little exercise will fail to achieve the results we want; too much will lead to over-training, leaving us stale and possibly leading ultimately to injury. The intensity and duration of exercise are dictated by the type of muscles we are using. The abdominal muscles work mainly to tense and hold the trunk steady during everyday activities. To do this, the muscles will require endurance, so that they can continue to work for long periods. This may be achieved by working the muscles at slightly less than half of their maximum strength. When the muscles contract, we try to build up the length of time they can hold the contraction until eventually we can hold the abdominal muscles tight for a duration of 30 seconds or so.

Where the abdominal muscles are used in sport, in addition to their role of supporting the trunk by holding it tight, they may be used in dynamic actions to move the trunk rapidly. In this case, the muscles must be trained for power and speed. It is important to note that the supporting (stabilising) function of the abdominal muscles is always re-trained first. Only when this has been achieved, and an athlete has good control of trunk alignment and movement, should power movements begin. The restoration of good support in the trunk forms the foundation upon which other types of training may be built.

The frequency of practice will change as we progress through the programme. This is because initially the intention is to learn correct exercise technique. When learning technique, we aim for a high number of short practice bouts to help concentration. For foundation movements most exercises are practised twice daily at first. The only exception is abdominal hollowing which is practised regularly throughout the day during everyday activities. Once the techniques of the exercises have been mastered, the number of practice bouts reduces and the exercises become harder (intensity increases). Harder exercise will require a longer recovery period, therefore exercises are practised every other day, with a full day in between to allow the muscles to recover.

The principle of training specificity

When a muscle is strengthened, its make-up actually changes. The muscle becomes larger and tighter, and there are alterations in the chemicals it contains. In addition, the way the brain controls the movement itself becomes smoother and more coordinated. All of these changes constitute what we call the *training adaptation*. In other words, the changes which the body makes are a direct result of the training itself. The exact adaptation will closely reflect the type of exercise which has been used, so we say that the muscle adaptation is 'specific' to the demands placed upon it.

An example from general sport may make this clearer. Imagine two people who run marathons. They want to reduce their times and go for a 'personal best'. If one person trains by running long distances and the other by running short sprints, who will be more successful in reducing their times? The answer is the person who runs distances. This type of training more accurately reflects the actions required during marathon running. Marathon runners need endurance. Short sprints will build mainly strength and speed and so, although the person using sprint training is getting fitter, the fitness is not the type required for the final marathon race. His body has changed (adapted) but these changes do not closely match those needed for running the marathon, they are not truly 'specific'.

Keypoint

For an exercise to be truly 'specific' it must closely match the action which we hope to improve.

When training the trunk muscles, the same principles of specificity apply. We need to know what function the trunk muscles perform and then tailor our training programme to improve this function. We have already seen that trunk muscle function falls broadly into two categories: support (stabilisation) and movement.

During stabilisation the trunk muscles work mainly isometrically (tense and hold) to make the trunk more solid. During movement, the muscles work concentrically and eccentrically to perform actions such as bending and twisting. Importantly, however, the trunk must be stable before more rapid movements can be attempted, and our training should take this into account.

Keypoint

The trunk muscles must be able to hold the spine effectively in a stable position before any vigorous trunk exercise is attempted.

With abdominal training we are aiming initially to restore the ability of the trunk muscles to stabilise the spine. Only when this has been achieved do we work on the muscles' ability to move the spine and provide power. For this reason, the initial part of the programme (foundation) works the muscles responsible for stability and re-trains their ability to tense and hold the trunk still. At this stage, if rapid movements such as sit-ups are used, they could actually damage the spine. Rapid actions are not specific to stabilisation and, until you are able to stabilise your spine and control it, rapid actions are dangerous.

Later, when stability has been re-trained, movements may begin. Initially they are slow and controlled, and later they build up speed and power. At this later stage, the movements practised mimic the actions used in sport. In this way the training remains specific to a subject's individual sport.

Keypoint

For effective abdominal training we must begin by improving spinal stability (core stability) and later move on to improve general movements.

Fitness components

Physical fitness may be defined as a person's ability to perform a physical task. Fitness may be seen on a continuum from an optimal level seen in the competitive athlete, through to the minimal standard required to stay healthy, and finally to a complete lack of fitness and the development of ill health (*see* fig. 3.1a). Fitness, then, is not simply a lack of disease, it is more than this; it is the ability of the body to allow a person to live a happy and well-balanced life.

We can think of fitness in two parts. There is *health-related* fitness, which involves items directly related to improving health and preventing disease. But also, there is task- or *performance-related* fitness which involves factors necessary for a person to perform a particular sport, or an activity at work, for example. To make things easier we can divide fitness into a series of components or 'S' factors (*see* fig. 3.1b).

- **Stamina** encompasses heart–lung fitness and also muscle endurance, or the ability to keep an exercise going.
- **Suppleness** (flexibility) and **strength** are both essential to the health of the joints.
- **Spirit** involves psychological factors which are important to both health and sport, such as motivation, how satisfied a person is with their own body, and a positive outlook on life.
- **Speed** (also encompassing power) is needed for explosive actions in sport.
- **Skill** is important to all actions, but especially those involving complex movements.
- **Specificity**, as we have seen, is important when matching exercise to sports actions.

The important point about the components of fitness is that they must be balanced. Often, exercise works on one component but not on others. For example, intensive bodybuilding may provide dramatic gains in strength, but

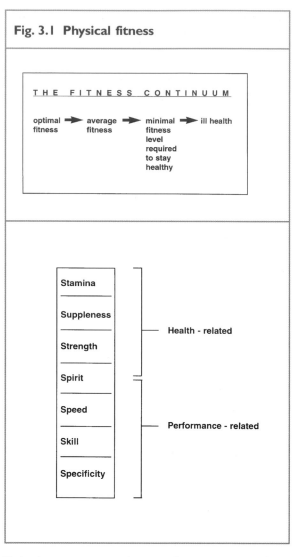

Fig. 3.1 Physical fitness

little improvement in suppleness or stamina. Running marathons will generate a high degree of stamina, but little suppleness or strength in the upper body.

When the fitness components become imbalanced, the body may be pulled out of alignment and injury can result. For example, if muscles are strong but not supple they will tend to pull or strain more easily. If a joint is too supple it will have little stability and may give way.

The aim with fitness is to improve all components more or less equally.

> ### Keypoint
> All the fitness components must be balanced for optimal health.

Building back fitness

We must differentiate between fitness of the whole body, and fitness of individual body components. Following the foundation movements in our abdominal training programme we aim to build *back fitness*. By this we mean the fitness components as they relate to the function of the back. For example, *stamina* is important to the back in two ways. Firstly, whole body stamina, simply because when a person is tired they are more likely to be injured. If you have a job which requires repeated use of your back, when you are tired you are open to injury. Secondly, stamina of the back muscles themselves. We use the back muscles to lift. If you perform 20 lifts, but your back muscle stamina is such that your muscles become fatigued after just 5 lifts, you are then open to injury for the remaining 15.

Suppleness within the sphere of back fitness reflects your ability to move unhindered. For example we have seen that to bend correctly you need to tilt your pelvis. The quantity of pelvic tilt is partially determined by hamstring length, so tight hamstrings will reduce your ability to bend and lift correctly. In the same way, you must have sufficient *strength* to lift, push or pull an object. You may need little back strength if you have a sedentary job, but if you work on a building site, your back strength has to be better than the heaviest weight you lift.

For each of the fitness components, when we are referring to back fitness we simply need to ask ourselves how a lack of particular components will impair our back function.

> ### Keypoint
> Back fitness refers to the way in which each fitness component effects back function.

Skill is often a fitness component which is forgotten. In the race to lift heavier weights, to stretch further or run faster, the quality of an exercise frequently takes a back seat to quantity. But as with so many things in life, more is not necessarily better. If the quality of a movement suffers, injury is more likely, because an action becomes clumsy. In the abdominal programme featured in this book we are aiming for *quality* of movement before quantity with every single exercise. The initial movements aim to re-educate the basic skills of spinal movement which have often lain dormant since childhood. This is essential because it forms the foundation for the whole programme. A person must be able to perform an exercise in a smooth, controlled fashion before the number of repetitions is increased.

> ### Keypoint
> The quality (control) of an exercise is more important than the quantity (number of repetitions) that can be performed.

Controlling the neutral spinal position

One of the most basic movements that you will need to control is pelvic tilting. You must be able to recognise when the pelvis tilts and pulls the spine out of alignment during everyday activities. As we have seen, the ideal alignment of the spine is a position where the pelvis is mid-way between being tilted fully back and fully forwards (*see* page 13). This is the *neutral position* and is where the joints, discs and tissues are subjected to loads they were designed to withstand. When we move away from the neutral position, stress on some tissues reduces, but stress on others increases dramatically. The neutral position is therefore a 'safety zone' for the spine.

The practical methods used to find the neutral position are covered elsewhere (*see* page 86). Once you have mastered the neutral position, use it regularly throughout the day and during all exercises. Try to sit in a chair with your spine in its neutral position. If you are in a gym using weight training apparatus, perform the exercise with your spine in its neutral position. When you are using stretching exercises, again try to keep the spine in its neutral position for as long as possible.

Keypoint

The spine is in its neutral position when the pelvis is level and the lower back is slightly hollow. Use the neutral position as often as possible to safeguard your back.

Progressive exercise

We have seen that to train the body we must overload it; that is, make the body work harder than it would normally during everyday activities. However, as fitness improves, the same amount of activity becomes easier and no longer taxes the body to the same degree. The training effect therefore reduces. To maintain the overload and continue to work the body sufficiently, the exercise must get harder as we become fitter. We now say that the exercise is progressing.

Keypoint

Over time, as an exercise becomes easier we must progress it (make it harder) to maintain the training effect.

One of the ways of progressing a weight training exercise is to perform a greater number of lifts (repetitions) with each training session. To progress stamina when running, we could simply run a longer distance with each training session. But there are other methods of progressing an exercise without increasing the amount of training that we do.

One method is to increase the degree of leverage on the body. In a sit-up action, for example, if the arms are held by the sides the weight of the upper body acts in the centre of the trunk, and the distance between the pivot point of the action (the hip joint) and the weight of the body represents a lever. If the arms are placed behind the head, their weight has moved away from the pivot point and so the leverage effect is greater. If the arms are held above the head, again the leverage has increased so the exercise has progressed (*see* fig. 3.2). In each case the weight of the body has obviously remained the same, but the increasing leverage effect has placed an additional overload on the working muscles.

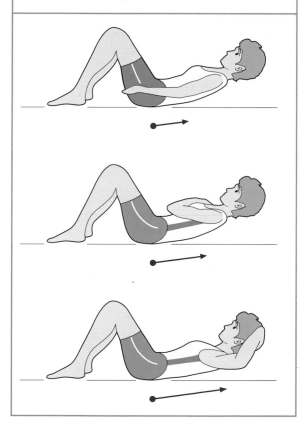

Fig. 3.2 Progressing an exercise using leverage. As the arms move higher up the body, the leverage distance between the hip and arm weight increases

A second method of exercise progression is to change the type of work a muscle has to perform. When a muscle is working against a load, for example when trying to lift a weight, it can work in three ways. If the muscle can create enough force to move the load, it is working concentrically. If it can only create enough force to hold the load still it is working isometrically. If it can't lift the weight or even hold it, but can make the weight lower more slowly, it is working eccentrically. An eccentric action is therefore easier than an isometric action and this, in turn, is easier than a concentric

action. If a muscle is very weak we should therefore begin with eccentric or isometric work (lowering or holding) before we move on to concentric work (lifting).

Adding resistance is another method of exercise progression for strength. The resistance may be anything which makes the movement harder. Elastic bands, springs, weights, and even the resistance of moving through water, will all strengthen muscle more effectively than free movement.

Targeting the deep muscle corset

To improve core stability we need to use firstly the deep corset muscles local to the spine – transversus, internal obliques and multifidus – and secondly the more general muscles which we have termed as 'global'. The abdominal programme in this book focuses on the local muscles first, and only when they are functioning normally do we begin to work the more general global muscles – in particular, the back and side back muscles (spinal extensors and quadratus lumborum), buttocks (gluteals), thigh muscles (quadriceps) and the powerful shoulder 'pulling' muscles (trapezius and rhomboids which retract the shoulder and latissimus dorsi). In each case, when working these powerful global muscles, alignment will be maintained by using the new-found core stability.

One of the reasons we focus on the deep muscle corset first is that these muscles may actually have forgotten how to work! If a person has suffered from back pain, or if they have had surgery where the tummy has been cut, the muscles may not work correctly. After pregnancy the muscles may take time to 'switch back on', and if a person is very overweight or very inactive, the muscles may not have been used for a long time. In each of these cases the deep muscle corset may not be functioning correctly and so we have to 'wake up' or 'switch on' the muscles before we can continue to train them with exercise.

Keypoint

Our abdominal programme must focus on getting the deep corset muscles working again, before other forms of exercise are used.

The transversus and internal oblique muscles pull the abdomen in. They do not bend the trunk as with a sit-up action. The sit-up action works the rectus muscle in the centre of the abdomen and the external obliques at the side. When these two powerful muscles work, they tend to dominate the movement and eclipse the action of the deep corset. To be able to restore the deep corset, therefore, the exercises must work these muscles in isolation. The action involves gently pulling the tummy button in, without bending the spine or moving the ribcage. For good core stability these muscles must also be able to hold themselves tight for a long period. Rather than building the exercise up and making it harder with weights or bands (resistance), for example, you gradually increase the time that the muscles can hold themselves tight (endurance). In a gym, an athlete may build up the arm muscles by gradually increasing the weight that is lifted, starting, for example, with 10 kg and moving up to 15 kg or 20 kg. This type of training is not suitable for the deep muscle corset. Instead, you tighten the muscles and initially hold them tight for 1 second, before gradually building up this holding time to 5 seconds or 10 seconds, all the time breathing normally and certainly not holding the breath.

Keypoint

To target the corset muscles rather than the 'sit-up' muscles, gently pull the tummy button in and hold the contraction, without bending the spine or moving the ribcage.

POSTURE

4

Posture is simply the relationship or alignment between the various parts of the body. It is important from two standpoints. Firstly, good posture underlies all exercise techniques. Your posture is really your foundation for movement. In the same way that a building will fall down if its foundations are shaky, your whole body will suffer if your posture is poor. Exercises which begin from the basis of poor posture tend to be awkward and clumsy. Because of this they are less effective and, more importantly, the person using awkward, clumsy movements is likely to be injured.

The second important point about posture is that an incorrect posture allows physical stress to build up in certain tissues, ultimately leading to pain and injury. For example, a person who is very round-shouldered may simply have started out with tightness in the chest muscles and weakness in the muscles which brace the shoulders back. If this combination had been corrected at the time, the poor posture may not have built up over the years. As a consequence of poor posture, the way that the joints move will change. Alteration in movement of this type will mean that joints can be subjected to uneven stresses. When this continues over the years, the eventual outcome can be the development of wear and tear (osteoarthritis) in later life.

Poor posture then gives two important features. Firstly joint alignment is not optimal so bodyweight, which would normally be distributed quite evenly across the joints, is taken more by one area than another (*see* fig. 4.1b). This leads to increased stress on portions of the joint. Secondly, good posture is one of balance and very little muscle work is actually needed

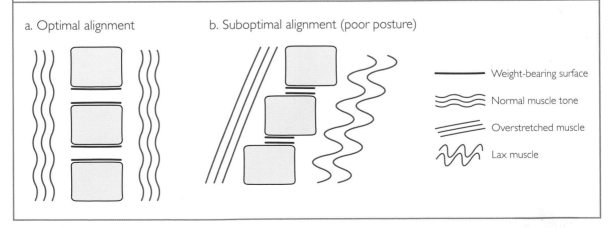

Fig. 4.1 Poor posture: increased stress on portions of the joint and muscles work harder because body segments are out of alignment (b)

a. Optimal alignment   b. Suboptimal alignment (poor posture)

Weight-bearing surface

Normal muscle tone

Overstretched muscle

Lax muscle

to maintain it. With a poor posture the muscles have to work much harder because the body segments are out of alignment (*see* fig. 4.1b). Increased muscle work of this type often leads to aching and the development of painful trigger points within the muscles.

> ### Keypoint
>
> With poor (sub-optimal) posture, stress on the joints is increased and the muscles have to work much harder.

We saw earlier that fitness is really a combination of various components which we called 'S' factors. In relation to posture, two of the most important fitness components are flexibility and strength. Postural changes are often associated with poor muscle tone (weakness) in some muscles together with too much tone (tightening) in others. This imbalance in tone gives an uneven pull from the muscles around a joint, and causes the joint to move off-centre (*see* fig. 4.2). Our aim with exercise is to redress the

balance in muscle tone by using stretching exercises to lengthen tight muscles, combined with strengthening exercises to increase the tone of lax muscles.

> ### Keypoint
>
> Your posture will affect the way you exercise, and the exercises you choose will in turn alter your posture.

Optimal posture

We cannot talk about a normal posture because very few people are 'normal' in the true sense of the word. Equally, if we talk about an average posture, the average may be very poor and this type of posture is far from ideal. Instead we should talk about an 'optimal' posture, where the various body segments are aligned correctly, and the minimum of stress is placed on the body tissues. This type of posture requires little

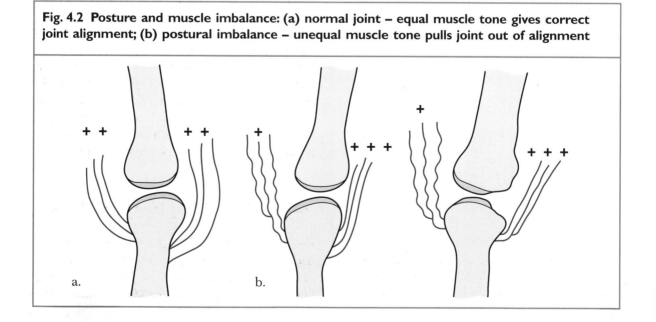

Fig. 4.2 Posture and muscle imbalance: (a) normal joint – equal muscle tone gives correct joint alignment; (b) postural imbalance – unequal muscle tone pulls joint out of alignment

a.

b.

muscle activity to maintain it because it is essentially balanced.

The various segments of the body work together like the links in a chain. Movement in one causes movement in the next link which is then passed on to the next, and so on. This means that a postural change in one part of the body can alter the alignment of another body part quite far away. Alterations in the feet are a good illustration of this point. Flat feet (*see* fig. 4.3), where the inner arch of the foot moves downwards, will in turn twist the shinbone and then the thighbone. Eventually these changes can be felt in the lower back, chest and neck. Because of this intimate link between body segments, it is important to correct any postural fault, however minor it may seem at the time.

Keypoint

In an optimal posture the body segments are correctly aligned, so very little effort is needed to maintain the position.

Fig. 4.3 Flat feet

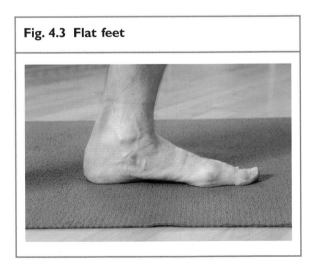

One method of looking at posture is to compare it to the posture line. In an optimal posture this line is similar to a plumb line dropped vertically

Fig. 4.4 Optimal posture: the lip of the pelvis forms a near-vertical line with the pubic bone in the groin

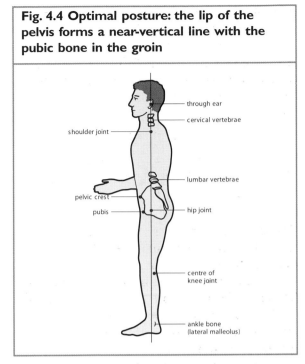

downwards from the top of the head. The body should be evenly distributed along this line (*see* fig. 4.4), and ideally the line should pass just in front of the knee joint, travel through the hip and shoulder joints and through the ear. Looking more closely at the pelvis, optimal pelvic alignment occurs when the front lip of the pelvis (anterior superior iliac spine) is in a direct vertical line with the pubic bone in the groin. In this position there should be a gentle curve to the lumbar spine and also to the neck. However, various alterations occur from this normal posture line which we need to consider.

Assessing your own posture

Before you can correct posture using the programme in this book, you must determine your current body alignment. Discovering your personal posture acts as a baseline **against** which to measure improvement as you go through the various exercises. You will need to work with a partner; they will assess your posture and you in turn will assess theirs. Ask your partner to stand against a straight vertical edge, such as a doorframe, or plumb line attached to a hook. Make sure that the edge of the line is slightly in front of their anklebone (lateral malleolus) and then compare their posture to this reference line. Fig. 4.4 shows the posture line, together with the optimal alignment. Photocopy this diagram, and then mark on the sheet the positions of their knee, hip, shoulder and ear. It is the centre point of each of these that we are interested in. The next step is to determine the position of your partner's pelvis. Draw an imaginary line from the furthest point forwards on the rim of their pelvis (anterior superior iliac spine) to their pubic bone. Determine whether this line is vertical or positioned at an angle.

Once you have assessed your partner's posture from the side, turn them around so that their back is towards you. Their feet should be about 10 cm (4 inches) apart. We will now continue the postural assessment using Table 4.1. Start by looking at their feet. The inner edge of the foot should have a gentle arch, and should not be flat. Moving up the leg, the Achilles tendon should be vertical and the bulk of the calf muscles (gastrocnemius and soleus) should be equal. The creases on the back of the knees (popliteal crease) and the lower edge of the buttocks (gluteal fold) should be on the same level for both sides of the body. The pelvis itself should be level horizontally and the spine aligned vertically. One of the ways that spinal alignment can be checked is to look at the skin creases on either side of the lower trunk; they should be equal in number and shape. The shoulder blades should be about three finger-breadths (6–8 cm) apart, and they should lie on the same horizontal line. The contours of the shoulders should be on the same level and they should

appear similar in size and shape. Finally, the head should be level and not tilted to one side. Record any changes from the optimal posture on a photocopy of Table 4.1.

The final method of posture assessment is to establish the depth of the curve in the lower back. Ideally, the curve should be gently hollow. When it is too deep, or too flat, the alignment of the lumbar region changes, indicating that the pelvic tilt is no longer correct. Assess the depth of the lumbar curve by standing with your back up against a wall. Stand with the feet 15–20 cm (6–8 inches) from the wall and the buttocks and shoulders touching the wall. Have your partner slide their hand between the wall and the small of your back. Ideally they should be able to push the hand through the gap only as far as the fingers. If the whole hand passes through, your lumbar curve is too deep. If they can only get the tips of the fingers between your back and the wall, the lumbar curve is too flat.

Summary

In an optimal posture:
- the hip, shoulder and ear lie in a vertical line;
- the pelvis is level;
- the lower spine should be gently hollowed;
- the inner edge of the shoulder blades are 6–8 cm (3 inches) apart.

General principles of postural exercise

To modify posture using exercise therapy, we must *stretch* tight muscle to allow correct movement to take place. If we simply try to exercise against a tight muscle it becomes self defeating – the exercise tries to move the body in one

Table 4.1	Assessing standing posture from behind			
Part of the body	**Changes**	**Part of the body**		**Changes**
Ear level/hair line 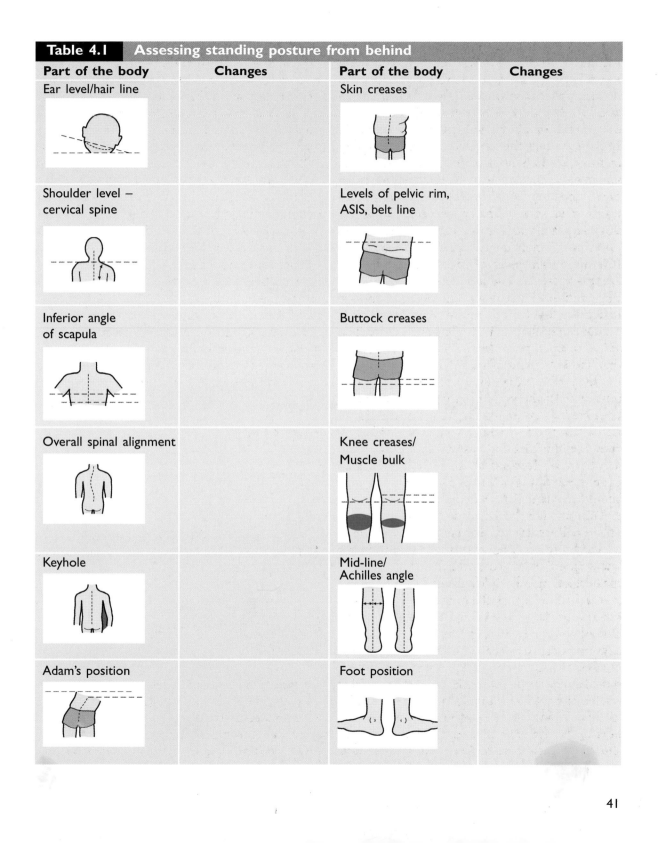		Skin creases		
Shoulder level – cervical spine		Levels of pelvic rim, ASIS, belt line		
Inferior angle of scapula		Buttock creases		
Overall spinal alignment		Knee creases/ Muscle bulk		
Keyhole		Mid-line/ Achilles angle		
Adam's position		Foot position		

direction and the body simply pulls back! Once we have stretched and free movement is possible, we now *shorten* lax muscle. This has the effect of holding the body part in the correct position. Stretching and strengthening (muscle shortening) in this way begins to correct the muscle imbalance which is usually the key feature of postural changes. However, changing the body tissues in this way will allow us to move correctly, but we still may not choose to do so. This is because the sub-optimal posture has been present for some time so it has become familiar – a bad habit if you like – hence the term *habitual posture*. To modify this, we must continually practise correct exercise postures so that we *rehearse* optimal posture and break our bad habits.

> ### Keypoint
>
> To modify sub-optimal posture we must (i) stretch shortened muscle (ii) strengthen/shorten lax muscle and (iii) rehearse correct posture and movement.

Hollow back posture

In an optimal posture the pelvis should be level, with the front rim of the pelvis and the pubic bone in a vertical line when viewed from the side. In this position, the lower part of the back (the lumbar spine) should be slightly hollowed. In the hollow back posture, however, the abdominal muscles become weak and lengthened, allowing the pelvis to

Fig. 4.5 Hollow back posture: (a) abdominal muscles sag; use the hip flexor stretch (b); and the lower back flexion stretch to correct it (c)

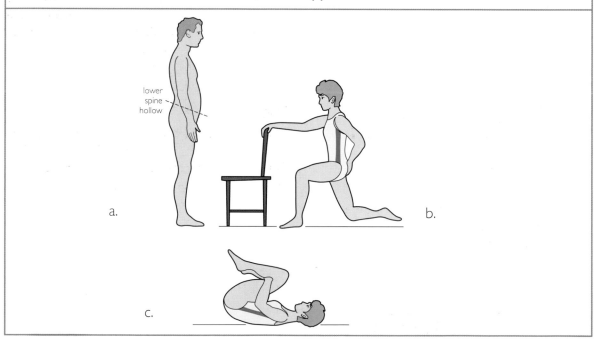

lower
spine
hollow

a.

b.

c.

tip forwards. When this happens the pull on the lumbar spine increases the lumbar curve. This increased curvature places stress on the discs and small joints (facet joints) of the lower spine. Over time, back pain can result. This can be particularly bad if a person stands for long periods.

The problem here is not abdominal strength but the *length* of the abdominal muscles, and the fact that the lower spine has been held in its hollow position for a long time. To correct the hollow back posture we must choose exercises which aim to shorten the abdominals. The abdominal hollowing exercises and trunk curl are the two which we use in the programme, and are described on pages 95 and 117 respectively. This type of posture is particularly common after pregnancy and is also seen in young female gymnasts, who choose this posture to walk.

The hollow back posture (*see* fig. 4.5a) is the classic 'beer belly' posture where many years of inactivity, combined with excess weight, leave the abdominals poorly toned. Often the angulation of the pelvis can shorten the hip flexor muscles (iliopsoas and rectus femoris) and these will require stretching. The key points of this posture which respond to exercise are:

- Tight hip flexors
- Anteriorly tilted pelvis
- Tight (extended) lumbar spine

Ex I Kneeling hip flexor stretch

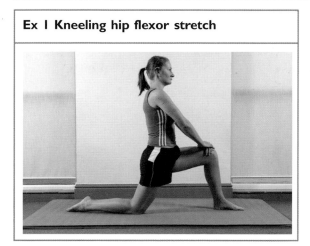

Starting position

Begin by kneeling on your right leg (half kneeling) with your left leg bent in front of you. Lightly tighten (tense) your abdominal muscles, breathing normally.

Action

From this position press your hips forwards, forcing the left (trailing) leg into extension.

Points to note

This exercise stretches the hip flexor muscles as they pass in front of the hip joint. However it will also press the ball of the hip socket (head of femur) forwards in its socket. In some cases this may cause pain. If so, it may indicate that the hip is anteriorly displaced (held forwards by tight tissue) and requires specialist treatment from a physiotherapist.

Training tip

It is essential that the lower spine does not hollow as you press your hips forwards. When this happens the movement is occurring at the lumbar spine rather than the hip.

Ex 2 Lower back flexion stretch

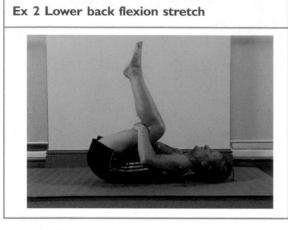

Starting position

Lie flat on the floor with your knees bent, and feet flat. This will have the effect of rounding the lower spine in the opposite direction to the hollow back.

Action

Grip your legs behind your knees and pull the knees in towards the chest. At the point where there is no further hip movement (the legs stop moving), pull in a little further so that your tailbone (sacrum and coccyx) lift from the mat.

Points to note

Some people have quite stiff hips, so the spine will begin to move when the knees are quite far from the chest. For others, the knees may have to be pulled right up onto the ribcage before the spine begins to move. The aim of the exercise is to tilt the pelvis and flex (round) the lower lumbar spine, posteriorly. The pulling action on the legs is therefore in and up.

Training tip

Make sure that the movement is slow and controlled. Never force the spine to move if it is stiff, but encourage it gently.

Abdominal muscle correction

Once you have stretched your hip flexor muscles and your lower back, you are ready to begin abdominal strengthening. To target the hollow back posture, begin with abdominal hollowing using exercise 18: abdominal hollowing standing (*see* page 94). When you are able to perform 10 repetitions of this exercise holding each contraction for 10 seconds (breathing normally), you can move on. To re-strengthen and shorten the abdominal muscles, use exercise 36: Trunk curl sequence (*see* page 117). Aim to perform 2 sets of 3 reps to begin with, and build up to 2 sets of 5–8 reps when you feel ready.

Head, neck and shoulder posture

Head and neck posture are important considerations when using abdominal exercises. Often standard sit-up movements, placing the hands behind the neck, can lead to the development of poor posture in this region and subsequent pain. In some cases this exercise can cause severe injury (*see* page 208).

When we look at a person from the side, their shoulder joint and ear should be positioned on the posture line. A common postural abnormality associated with the upper spine is called the round back posture (*see* fig. 4.6b). Changes occur in the position

Fig. 4.6 Round back posture: (a) normal; (b) incorrect head and shoulder alignment

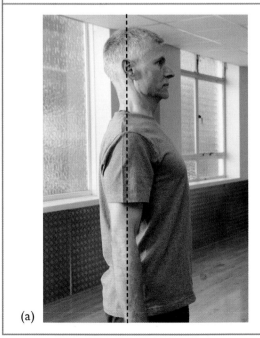
(a)

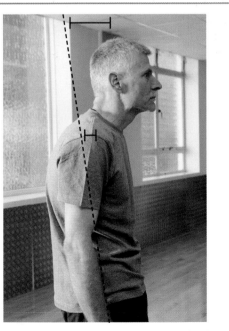
(b)

of the head and neck, the shoulder joint and upper (thoracic) spine. The normal curve of the thoracic region is lost and pain often develops between the shoulder blades.

When we look at a person from the side, if they have the round back posture, the head is often held forwards with the shoulders being excessively rounded. The chest muscles (pectorals) are normally too tight, while the muscles that pull the shoulders back (retractors) are often too weak. Looking at the person from the back, the shoulder blades should be roughly 6–8 cm (3 inches) apart.

However, in the round back posture, weakness of the shoulder muscles allows the shoulder blades to drop apart and to twist.

The key points of the round back posture which respond to exercise therapy are:
- Tight/short chest muscles
- Lax shoulder retractors
- Rounded upper spine (flexed)
- Head held forwards (protracted)
- Shoulder blades too far apart (abducted)

Ex 3 Chest stretch in room corner

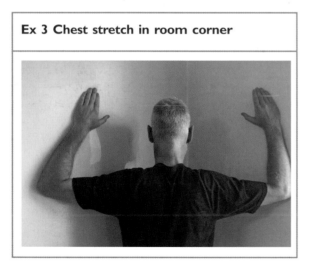

Starting position

Begin standing in the corner of a room with your upper arms horizontal and forearms vertical. Place one forearm on each wall.

Action

Slowly lean forwards. Press your chest into the corner of the room.

Points to note

This exercise places stress on the shoulder joint itself. Normally this is not a problem, but if you have ever dislocated your shoulder, do not use this action unless you are supervised by a physiotherapist.

Training tip

If you find this stretch very hard, take up a lunge position (one foot in front of the other) so that less of your bodyweight is taken on your shoulders.

Ex 4 Chin tuck and hold

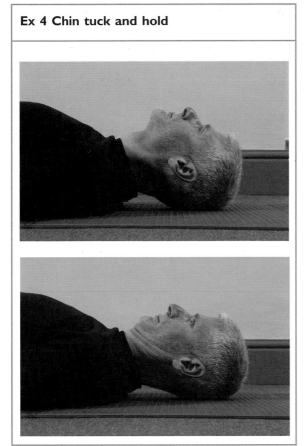

Starting position

Begin lying on the floor. If your head tilts backwards, place a folded towel beneath it.

Action

Tuck your chin in as though trying to place it into the top of your breastbone (sternum). Hold the inward position for 5–10 seconds, breathing normally.

Points to note

There is very little movement in the action, but you should feel a slight stretch at the top of your neck (sub-occipital region).

Training tip

If your neck is very stiff, you can place a little pressure on your chin with your fingers. Try this for 2–3 repetitions before you hold for 5–10 seconds.

Ex 5 Shoulder brace

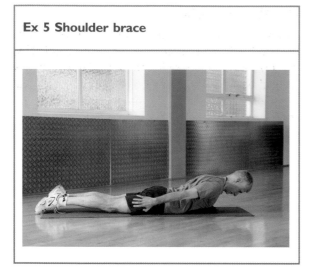

Starting position

Lie on the floor with your arms by your sides and a thin cushion or folded towel beneath your chest.

Action

Gently tighten your abdominal muscles and draw you shoulder blades together slightly. Lift first your arms, and then your head and chest from the floor. Hold the lifted position for 2–3 seconds and then lower slowly.

Points to note

The tightening action of the abdominal muscles and shoulder blades (scapulae) stabilises both your lower (lumbar) and upper (thoracic) spine during this exercise. You only need to lift high enough for your chest to clear the ground. Do not over-arch your back.

Training tip

Imagine the top of your head is being pulled to the far wall as you lift. This will help you lengthen your spine rather than over-arching it.

Ex 6 Thoracic spine stretch over roll

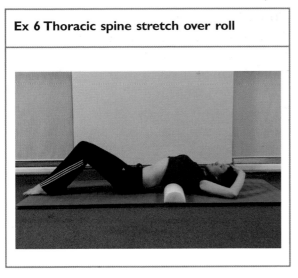

Starting position

Begin lying on the floor with a rolled towel or foam roller placed crossways beneath your upper back. Lightly tighten your abdominal muscles by drawing them inwards.

Action

Breathe normally and, with each breath out (expiration), try to relax over the roll to encourage your spine to be pressed flat (extension). Lie in this position for 2–3 minutes.

Points to note

There may be very little movement available, especially if your spine is very tight. Initially this position may be quite uncomfortable, but this should subside in about 30 seconds as your muscles relax. If you feel pain which increases, stop the exercise and consult a physiotherapist.

Training tip

If you find you head tips back, place a folded towel beneath your head. If you find your back hollows excessively, bend your knees.

Swayback posture

We have seen that to assess posture we compare a person's body alignment to a vertical plumb line. In the swayback posture, the pelvis stays level but the hips move forwards of the posture line (*see* fig. 4.7). Because the hip joint now lies in front of the posture line, the hip is effectively pulled backwards into extension. In this position the hip flexor muscles are lengthened, exactly the opposite situation to that which we saw in the hollow back posture earlier (*see* page 42).

If we compare the normal and swayback postures, we can see that in a normal posture the furthest point forwards is the chest, while the furthest point backwards is the buttocks. In the swayback, however, the furthest point forwards is the abdomen, and the thoracic spine is the furthest point back. Looking at the lower back in the normal posture, the lumbar curve is gently hollow along its whole length. In the swayback, however, the hollow is sharp and more pronounced in the lower region of the spine. Finally, in the normal posture the spine and leg are close to the posture line, but in the swayback the spine and leg form a curve with the person's whole body profile taking on the shape of a letter 'V' turned on its side. The swayback is a relaxed or slumped posture frequently seen in adolescents.

Correction of the swayback posture is accomplished through the practice of correct body alignment, rather than specific strength or stretching exercises. Because the bodyline in the swayback is curved, a person with this posture appears shorter. Simply by trying to stand tall, and lengthen the whole body while activating both the abdominal muscles (lumbar stabilisors) and shoulder blades (thoracic stabilisors), the swayback can be corrected over time.

Keypoint

The keypoints of the swayback posture which respond to exercise therapy are:

- Pelvis and hips move forwards
- Body height reduces
- Reduced postural muscle tone

Fig. 4.7 Swayback posture

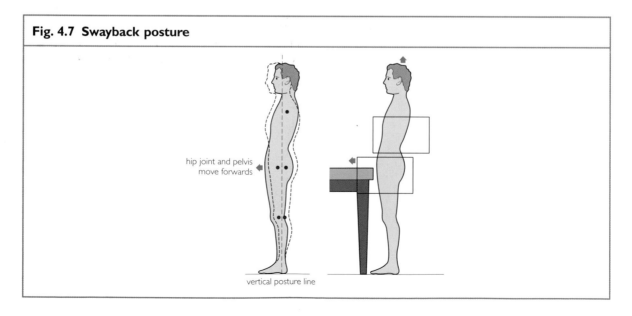

hip joint and pelvis move forwards

vertical posture line

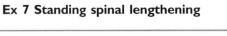

Ex 7 Standing spinal lengthening

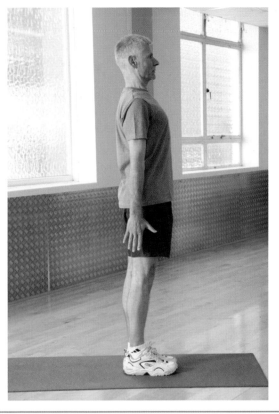

Starting position

This exercise comes from yoga, where it is called the mountain pose (tadasana). Begin standing, with your feet together, and hands by your sides.

Action

Work from the floor upwards in a sequence. Lift your inner ankles slightly, correcting any tendency to flatten your feet. Tighten your thigh muscles (quadriceps) and draw your legs together (hip adductors). Pull your tummy in slightly and draw your tailbone downwards, correcting any tendency to over-arch your spine. Draw your shoulder blades together slightly and downwards (adduction and depression) and finally tuck your chin in.

Points to note

Each of these movements is very slight, tightening the posture muscles in turn. Take care not to tense too much or hold your breath.

Training tip

Reach the crown of your head to the ceiling and the tips of your fingers to the floor.

Ex 8 Low back extension stretch

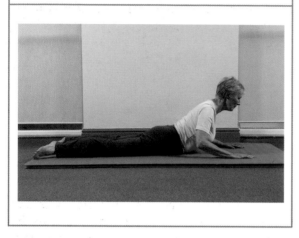

Starting position

Begin lying on the floor with your arms bent and hands by your sides – the 'press-up' position.

Action

Press with your hands and lift your chest from the floor keeping your hips down. Push for 5 seconds, and then hold the upper position for 5 seconds and then lower.

Points to note

If your spine is very tight, you may not be able to lift very high. By repeating the action, however, you should find that your lower back becomes more flexible.

Training tip

If you have very little movement, you will find it easier on your arms to place your hands further forwards on the mat.

Flatback posture

In the flatback posture, a person shows a markedly reduced lumbar curve. When standing straight with the spine up against a wall, you should normally be able to place the flat of your hand between the wall and your lower spine. Someone with a flatback posture may only be able to place one or two fingers in the gap formed. In this posture, the pelvis has tilted backwards and the lumbar spine has been pulled with it. The flatback is commonly seen where a person has spent a lot of time sitting slumped in a chair. It is particularly common after a bout of back pain where a person has rested in bed for too long. Stiffness may occur either when bending forwards or bending backwards, with the spine becoming almost fixed in the flatback position.

The flatback can also occur following repeated abdominal work involving flexion alone, such as crunches without performing spinal extension work to move the spine in the opposite direction. This is seen with inexperienced bodybuilders aiming for a 'six pack' who make the mistake of simply performing more and more reps in a single movement, creating a postural imbalance.

Stretching can help to alleviate the pain from this condition, providing it is performed gently to encourage movement rather than to force it. The stretching should feel slightly uncomfortable because the exercises are working on very tight structures. However, they should not give back pain and, in cases where this occurs, exercise should only be carried out under the supervision of a physiotherapist.

> ## Keypoint
>
> The keypoints of the flatback posture which respond to exercise therapy are:
> - Lumbar curve (lordosis) flattened
> - Lower (lumbar) back tight

Functional movements of the spine

A functional movement is one which occurs in normal day-to-day activities rather than in the gym. Functional movements are important because they represent the situation in which your abdominal muscles will actually work. For example, if you perform an ankle exercise on a machine in the gym, you will build up your calf muscles. This is not a functional movement, however, because, apart from in the gym, this is not a situation that you would use in day-to-day life. You will use your calf muscles when you walk, run, and jump. For this reason the functional movement most useful for the lower limb is gait (walking and running), and variations on gait movements can be adapted as functional lower limb exercise.

For the abdominal muscles, one of the most important functional movements is bending and lifting. If the abdominal muscles are not working to stabilise the spine correctly in this movement, excessive stress is imposed on the area and low back pain is frequently the result.

Once we have determined your body alignment when you are still (posture), the next step is to look at body alignment in functional movement related to the back. For this we must study the lifting mechanism.

The lifting mechanism

To illustrate the lifting mechanism, let's take an analogy of the spine as a fishing rod. When we lift a fish on the end of a fishing rod we are lifting a weight (the fish) using the power of our hands. To be able to do this the fishing rod itself acts as a lever which is both flexible, but strong. If it were very weak like a piece of old rope, the fishing rod wouldn't be an effective lever and we would be unable to lift the fish. In this case, the lever is not able to transmit the force created by our hands.

This is exactly what happens to our spine when lifting. We lift any heavy object by providing power from our buttock (gluteal) muscles. This power is transmitted along our spine acting as a lever. This only works if our spine is strong. If it is weak or 'unstable' it cannot transmit the force created by our powerful gluteal muscles. Following back pain, this is precisely what we see. Someone who has chronic low back pain often has very poor buttock muscles and a weakened and unstable spine. They cannot create sufficient force from their buttock muscles so they try to lift instead with their back muscles. The result is that these muscles become strained and go into painful spasm. The answer is to train for stability of the spine and build up the gluteal muscles – precisely what we will do later in this book.

Check out your lifting posture

Good alignment is a key to spinal health, and lifting is no exception. To minimise stress on the spine and reduce the likelihood of injury, a good lifting posture is essential. The power for the lift should come from your legs. Bend the knees, and use the powerful gluteal muscles and hamstrings. If your gluts are weak, you may have a tendency to lock your legs out straight and use your back muscles instead. This causes your back to bend and you lose the normal inward curve (lordosis) in your lower spine. The rounded posture travels the whole way up the spine and you will get round shoulders and tend to look down. Finally, if core stability is poor your abdominal muscles will be weak and lax.

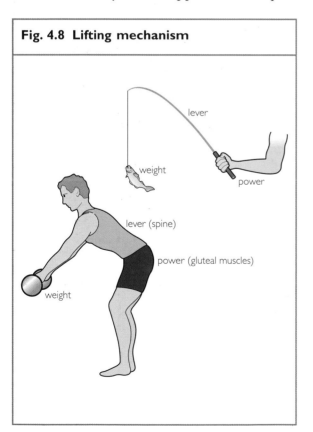

Fig. 4.8 Lifting mechanism

lever

weight

power

lever (spine)

power (gluteal muscles)

weight

Table 4.2	Lifting posture
Good	Bad
• Knees bent	• Knees locked out straight
• Gluteal muscles toned and powerful	• Gluteals flattened and wasted
• Low back hollow (lordosis)	• Low back bent (lordosis reversed)
• Abdomen tight and hollow	• Abdomen lax and 'pot belly'
• Shoulders braced (scapular setting)	• Shoulders rounded (scapular abduction)
• Head looking forwards	• Head looking down
• Object held close to body	• Object held at arms length

Fig. 4.9 Lifting posture

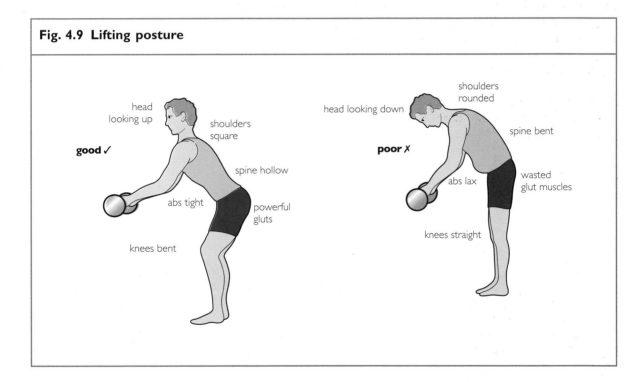

Ex 9 The hip hinge

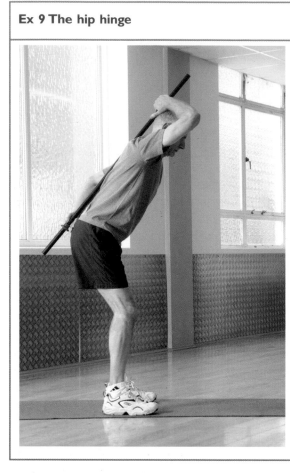

Prior to using this exercise, practise exercise 18: abdominal hollowing in standing, page 94, first.

Starting position

Begin by standing with your feet hip-width apart. Hold a stick along the length of your spine so that you have three points of contact – tailbone (sacrum and coccyx), upper (thoracic) spine, and head resting on the stick. Gently tighten (hollow) your abdominal muscles as in exercise 18: abdominal hollowing in standing.

Action

Bend your knees and hips, and angle your spine forwards to 45 degrees, keeping your three points of contact with the stick at all times.

Points to note

If you allow your back to bend, you will notice your head moving off the stick (upper spine rounding), or your tail moving off the stick (lower spine rounding).

Training tip

Rather than bending forwards, think about pointing your tail to the wall. This visualisation encourages a tipping (hip flexion) rather than bending (spine flexion) action of the spine.

DIET AND EXERCISE

5

People often begin using abdominal exercises in the hope of reducing their waistline; they join a local gym or exercise class and work hard for many months. Eventually, however, they can lose enthusiasm if they fail to see the results they want. Instead of reducing their waistline all they have achieved is a marginal re-shaping, and they give up exercising, disillusioned. There are two reasons for the failure of this type of training. Firstly, if exercise is not coupled with a correct diet, you will not lose significant amounts of weight. Secondly, the type of training will determine the effect it has on your waistline. The wrong type of training will often have little effect at all.

Bodyweight and body fat

People often talk about being overweight, meaning that they have too much loose flesh around the abdomen (men), and around the abdomen, thighs and buttocks (women). However, your bodyweight is made up of a number of things; bone, muscle, fluids, body organs, fat and other tissues all contribute to your total weight. Take a sauna and you will lose weight because you sweat water, but this is not a permanent weight loss. Begin a weight training programme and your muscles will become sleek, firm and toned. This may be desirable, but because muscle weighs more than fat you may actually gain a few pounds. What we really mean when we say someone is overweight is that they have too much fat, which is possibly linked to flabby muscle.

Body fat occurs in different types. *Essential* body fat is found around the body organs and within the marrow in the centre of the bones. Women have more fat than men because they carry additional *sex-specific* fat which is important for a variety of hormonal functions. If the level of fat is reduced too much, as can be the case in young girls who diet excessively, for example, a woman's periods will often stop due to the hormonal changes caused by the low body fat. The other type of fat is storage fat which is found beneath the skin and acts as a depot for energy. It is the *storage* fat which often becomes excessive.

In order to lose inches from the waistline we need to reduce the amount of body fat, while maintaining a healthy, balanced diet, but this must be coupled with exercise to tone and shape the muscles of the abdomen or they will remain flabby.

Keypoint

The amount of body fat you have is more important than your weight.

Obesity

Obesity is simply an excessive amount of fat in the body. The World Health Organisation

Table 5.1	Body mass index (BMI)	
BMI (kg/m²)		**Category**
• Less than 18.5		• Underweight
• 18.5 – 24.9		• Normal weight
• 25.0 – 29.9		• Overweight
• 30.0 – 39.9		• Obese
• More than 40.0		• Severely obese

(WHO) defines obesity in terms of body mass index or BMI, saying that a person with a BMI over 30 is obese (*see* table 5.1). BMI is calculated by dividing a person's weight in kilograms (kg) by their height in metres squared (m²). So, for example, if you weigh 70 kg (155 lb) and are 1.82 m (6.0 ft) tall, your BMI is 70 divided by 1.82 squared (3.3) which is 21. Looking at table 5.1 we see that a BMI of 21 is within the normal weight section.

Although BMI is a useful measure, it does not take into account the ratio of lean tissue (muscle) to fat (adipose tissue). As a consequence, BMI values can overestimate body fat in athletes who are very muscular, and underestimate it in those who are frail or wasted, especially the elderly. For this reason age, sex, body type, and race (ethnicity), should also be considered.

From the point of view of cardiovascular risk factors especially, where the body fat is stored is important. *Central obesity*, where body fat is concentrated around the middle of the body, is more dangerous than *general obesity* where the fat is evenly distributed all over the body. This is because central obesity sees body fat stored around the organs (visceral fat) resulting in a 'beer belly' appearance. This type of fat can change the concentration of the hormone insulin in the blood and is an important factor in the development of diabetes. If excessive, central obesity is obvious, but clinically its presence is determined by waist measurement and waist-hip ratio. Central obesity is present when the waist measurement is greater than 102 cm (40 inches) in men and 88 cm (35 inches) in women, and the waist-hip ratio is greater than 0.9 and 0.85 for men and women respectively.

Keypoint

In central obesity, fat is stored around the body organs. The condition is important in the development of diabetes.

The rapid rise in obesity during the last 25 years is due to a combination of factors, the two most important being diet and lack of exercise (sedentary lifestyle). The consumption of energy- (calorie-) dense fast food has tripled in the Western world during the last quarter of the 20th century. A sedentary lifestyle fails to burn off these excessive calories, and it is both general activity as well as exercise which is important here. For example, the school run (driving children to school rather than encouraging them to walk) is thought to be a prime mover in the development of childhood obesity. That small walk to and from school may not seem much but, because it is regular, it is a vital

Keypoint

The most important factors in the development of obesity are (i) over consumption of energy rich foods and (ii) a sedentary lifestyle.

amount of exercise in an otherwise predominantly sedentary Western world.

The feeding control mechanism

One of the main factors which assists in the control of an ideal bodyweight is the feeding control mechanism (FCM). This is situated within the brain in an area called the *hypothalamus*. The FCM controls bodyweight by matching the amount of energy obtained from food to the requirements of the body through activity. If the amount of energy going into the body is exactly equal to the amount going out, the bodyweight will remain constant. Individuals who are overweight tend to have lost the ability to match their energy requirements to their diet. Unless the FCM is re-set, long-term control of an ideal bodyweight is unlikely. One of the problems with crash diets is that although they lead to a short-term reduction in weight, because they restrict the amount of energy going in, the FCM tries to conserve energy and the 'tick-over speed' of the body (the 'basal metabolic rate') is slowed by as much as 45 per cent. This means that weight loss will slow down and a person can quickly lose motivation because they always desire more food than they are getting. When they stop the diet, the weight goes back on and we get a yo-yo effect of repeated weight loss and weight gain over a period of time. A more effective method of weight control is to combine good dietary habits with regular activity as this type of

Keypoint

Combining a high-quality diet with regular activity is the key to achieving and maintaining an ideal body size.

programme has been shown to re-set the FCM to the correct levels.

Calories

The energy taken into the body as food, and that expended during activity, is measured in calories, a measure of the heat a food would produce if it were burnt. One kilocalorie or Calorie (with a capital 'C') is the more common measure, and this is equivalent to 4.2 joules, the joule being the other measure of food energy seen on food packaging. Some of the main constituents of food are *carbohydrate*, a starchy or sugary material giving energy; *fat*, an energy store and *protein*, used to build the body tissues. All of these substances can be used by the body for energy, and so may be measured in Calories. Both carbohydrate and protein produce the same amount of energy. Fat is a more concentrated energy source, and can produce more than double the energy of the other two types of foods. This is why fat is used as an energy store, and reducing it in the diet is a good way to lose weight. Another source of energy is alcohol which has almost the same number of Calories as fat.

Foods are made up of a mixture of nutrients, and so we give each food a total Calorie value, reflecting the proportional amounts of the various nutrients it contains. The Calorie value is useful when the food is used as part of a Calorie-controlled diet to lose weight, but does not relate to the quality of the food. This is because high-Calorie foods are not necessarily high in vitamins and minerals, and fibre contains virtually no Calories at all, but is still an important part of the diet.

Energy is used up by the body in two ways. Even without movement, the body has a certain 'resting energy' requirement for breathing, the heartbeat, digestion and other bodily functions.

The amount of energy needed for these processes can vary from person to person depending on many factors, including body size. This resting energy is the *basal metabolic rate*, and normally uses up about 1200 Calories each day. The other requirement for energy comes from 'voluntary activity', including things such as manual work and exercise. People who have active jobs, and those who exercise intensely, will burn up more Calories.

Different sports will burn off Calories at different rates. For example, slow jogging may use 120 Calories an hour, while driving a car needs only 48 Calories. Intense swimming or circuit weight training, where all the muscles are worked, can use over 250 Calories in the same time. In order to burn Calories significantly, the exercise should be continuous for 20–30 minutes and must be practised regularly.

Losing weight

When the amount of energy taken into the body from food equals the amount being expended during exercise and everyday activities, a person is in *energy balance*. In this situation they will neither gain nor lose weight. If the energy input is greater than the expenditure, the extra energy will be stored as fat. If too little energy is taken in, the body makes up the deficit by drawing on stored energy and burning up fat.

Clearly, one method of losing weight is simply to eat less. However, this has a number

of disadvantages for those exercising regularly. Firstly, it is more difficult to eat a sufficient quantity of nutrients; secondly, tissue other than fat is lost, particularly with extreme weight loss diets. At the onset of a diet, 70 per cent of weight loss is from water (*see* fig. 5.1), reducing to about 20 per cent by the time a person has been dieting for two weeks. Fat loss speeds up as the diet is continued, changing from 25 per cent of the total weight loss in the early days of a diet, to about 70 per cent after two weeks. Protein loss increases from 5 per cent to 15 per cent in the same timescale.

Rather than crash dieting then, a better method is to improve the general quality of the diet. It is not just the amount of food, but the type of food which is important. High-energy foods (those with a lot of Calories, especially

Keypoint

When the amount of energy coming into your body as food equals the amount going out through activity and exercise, you are said to be in 'energy balance'.

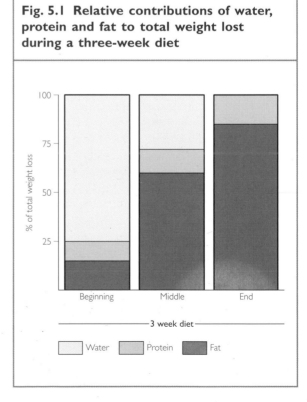

Fig. 5.1 Relative contributions of water, protein and fat to total weight lost during a three-week diet

fat and alcohol) should be restricted, and these should be replaced with low-Calorie equivalents. The total amount of food may remain the same. It is important not to reduce the carbohydrate foods too much as these provide both the energy for exercise and necessary amounts of fibre. It is more important to reduce the high-fat foods, for a low-fat/high-carbohydrate diet.

The essential items to restrict are alcohol, fast foods such as chips (French fries) and crisps (potato chips), and snacks such as chocolate, because these are high in fat. Trim all visible fat and grill, rather than fry, food. Use less refined foods such as wholemeal bread and cereals, and eat starchy foods such as potatoes and pasta, rather than sweet foods, for energy.

Glycemic load

Substances from digested food are converted to blood sugar (glucose) and transported from the digestive system to the muscles and other body cells where they are used to release energy. Despite the fact that we don't eat continually, the level of blood sugar remains fairly constant at about 90mg/100ml (5mM). Too much blood sugar (hyperglycemia) or too little (hypoglycemia), if it occurs over time, can create health problems. The most common condition is *diabetes mellitus* which is persistent hyperglycemia. Several hormones are responsible for maintaining a constant level of blood sugar, the most important being *insulin*, which reduces blood glucose.

If you eat food which raises the blood sugar too much, your body will produce insulin to lower it again. However, if blood sugar is too high it can damage your blood vessels, making it harder for insulin to work. To compensate, your body simply produces more insulin and you are said to be *insulin resistant*. Eventually, your blood sugar will fall, but it does so rapidly, and your energy level plummets. You feel lethargic and crave food again. Keeping blood sugar constant is the key, because it stops the yo-yo effect of energy going up and down taking your appetite with it. More constant blood sugar means a regular supply of available energy and no hunger pangs!

Glycemic index (GI) is a measure of the effect of carbohydrates in food on blood sugar level. Foods that break down quickly (fast releasing) and give a sudden surge in blood sugar have a high GI, and those that break down more slowly (slow releasing), and give a gradual and controlled increase in blood sugar, have a low GI. In general, foods with a lower GI are healthier (less refined wholefoods or *slow foods*) and those with a high GI less healthy (more refined *fast foods*).

A small amount of high GI food could give the same change in blood sugar as a large amount of low GI food, so most authorities now recommend using glycemic load or GL which is a combination of both glycemic index and portion size.

For a healthy diet, we should be aiming to eat lower GL foods to maintain a level blood sugar, and eating no more than 40–50 GL units per day split over three meals (10–12 GL each) and two snacks (5 GL each). Table 5.2 shows some high and low GL foods. The full international table of glycemic index and glycemic load from the American Journal of Clinical Nutrition (2002) is available at http://www.ajcn.org/cgi/reprint/76/1/5.pdf. This table lists over 700 foods!

Keypoint

The hormone insulin reduces blood sugar (glucose) and is important in diabetes.

> **Keypoint**
>
> Glycemic index (GI) is a measure of the effect a food has on blood sugar level. Glycemic load (GL) combines portion size with glycemic index.

Looking at these tables, you can see that food choices are very important. If you choose a bowl of cornflakes, toast and butter and a cup of sweet tea you will have had a high GL breakfast and, although you will feel full, your energy level will dip mid-morning leaving you craving a chocolate bar. A bowl of porridge, some fresh fruit and a herbal tea will be low GL, releasing its energy far more slowly. Your energy level will be maintained at a more constant level leaving your appetite satisfied for the whole morning. Similarly a tuna mayonnaise baguette for lunch is a higher GL choice that a tuna salad with a couple of oat cakes.

Can exercise help you to lose weight?

There are a number of myths about exercise and weight loss which we need to dispel. It is often said that if you start exercising your appetite will increase and you will put on weight. This is not so. Regular exercise helps to re-set the feeding control mechanism. Studies have shown that those who exercise regularly have a greater ability to match the amount of food they want with the amount their body actually needs. This is especially important in children. Scientific studies have consistently shown that inactive children are more likely to be overweight in later life.

Table 5.2	Glycemic load (GL) of some common foods per serving
Food	**GL value**
Baguette	15
Oatcakes	8
Banana	10
Carrots	3
Apple	6
Muesli	10
Cornflakes	21
Porridge	2
Tortilla	12
Potato	9
Potato crisps	11
White rice	15
Melon	3

A second myth concerns the ability of exercise to burn off fat. You will hear people say that you would have to exercise all day to burn off the pounds they need to lose. After all, to lose just 0.45 kg (1 lb) of bodyweight you would have to chop wood for 10 hours or play volleyball for 32 hours! However, this type of argument fails to take into account the regularity of exercise. Although only a small number of Calories are burned with each exercise bout, the cumulative effect is great. If, for example, you were to play two hours of golf, it would take four to five weeks to burn off 0.45 kg of fat. But, if you play each week for the whole year, you will have burnt off over 6 kg (nearly a stone) in total – a very significant amount!

Coupling exercise with a good diet is the best route to permanent weight loss. As mentioned, exercise helps to re-set the FCM, and the desire to eat too much is reduced. Secondly, exercise speeds up the metabolic rate – the 'tick over' of the body – so that even when exercise has finished, energy will continue to be burned off. A half-hour workout, for example, will continue to burn up Calories for three or four hours afterwards. Of course, exercise will not only reduce weight but will also increase muscle tone and add greatly to the overall improvement in physical appearance.

Body type

People often compare themselves to others to determine if they are satisfied with their body. Are they too big or too small, too fat or too thin? Is their waistline OK? Are their hips too big? Although this is understandable, one of the problems is that we each have a different body type. In other words, your body is unique, and

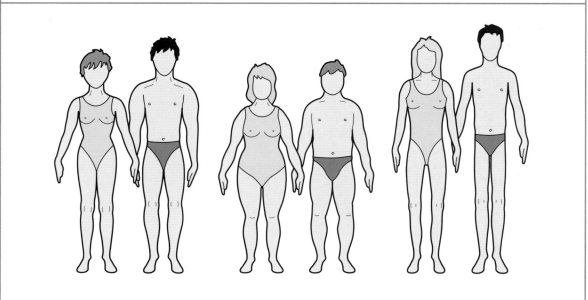

Fig. 5.2 Body types: (left) mesomorph – muscular; (centre) endomorph – rounded; (right) ectomorph – linear

the only way to judge if you are in good shape is to know what feels and looks good for you.

The shape of the human body can be classified into three distinct body types or *somatotypes* (*see* fig. 5.2). The first type is angular (*mesomorph*). This type of body tends to be muscular, with a typical 'Tarzan' appearance: the shoulders are broad and the waist is slim. These people tend to have large bones and thick-set muscles. The second type is more rounded (*endomorph*) and represented by the 'Billy Bunter' shape. These individuals have a smooth, soft outline with a 'pear drop' appearance. The waist and chest are often roughly the same measurement, and fat is carried on the upper arms and thighs as well as around the waist. The third type is linear (*ectomorph*) represented by the typical 'bean poles'. These individuals tend to be tall and thin, with long legs and arms. Their muscles are long and fine, and they have a wiry appearance.

In reality, we are all a mixture of these three extremes. But the proportion of each body type you have will determine your overall shape, and there is little you can do to change this.

Take as an example a young girl with a very rounded, stout appearance. She sees models in the fashion magazines who are tall and thin with long delicate limbs. Wanting to change her appearance she joins a local aerobics class and starts dieting. Initially her weight reduces, but she becomes unhappy because she feels she is not achieving what she wanted. She is fitter, and her muscles are more toned, but she does not look like the magazine models? Why? Not because she has failed to work hard enough, but because she has a different body type. She has a mixture of the rounded (endomorph) and angular (mesomorph) physiques, while the magazine model has a linear (ectomorph) body type. This young girl is now fit and toned. She should be happy, energetic and carefree.

Instead she is depressed and self-conscious because she is aiming to change the body type she was born with. This is impossible. It is far better to achieve the best you can for your own body than to want someone else's!

Keypoint

Our bodies combine tendencies towards being fat, lean and muscled. The combination of these factors you were born with determines your body type.

Summary

- Body fat is a more important consideration than bodyweight. This includes muscle, bone, tissues and fluids as well as fat.
  - Body mass index (BMI) is calculated by dividing a person's weight in kilogrammes (kg) by their height in metres squared (m^2).
- The feeding control mechanism (FCM) in the brain attempts to match the amount of energy you take in as food to the amount you burn off through physical activity.
- Starches and sugars are energy-providing foods called carbohydrates. Fat is an energy store and is high in Calories.
- Your basal metabolic rate (BMR) is the 'tick-over rate' of your body. Exercise increases this, re-activates your FCM, and increases muscle tone.
  - Low GL foods are better for health and help you to lose weight.
  - Keeping your blood sugar more constant by focusing your diet on low GL is a good health investment.
- You cannot change the body type you were born with.

COMMON ABDOMINAL EXERCISES

6

One of the aims of this book is to improve the standard of abdominal exercises by making exercises for this body part both safer and more effective. To fulfill this aim, the first thing we need to do is to take a close look at some commonly practised exercises and see where these go wrong. Although these exercises have been practised for many years in numerous gyms and exercise classes, there is still much room for improvement.

The sit-up

The sit-up is often the first exercise approached when abdominal training is considered. Unfortunately this exercise has a number of inherent dangers, especially for the spine. By knowing what happens to the body during this action we can reduce these dangers considerably.

Begin the exercise lying flat on your back. As soon as you lift your head from the floor, the abdominal muscles begin to work. This is because the muscles lifting the neck pull on the ribcage. To stop the ribs from moving, and hold them firm, the abdominal muscles must tighten. As the exercise continues, you begin to lift your trunk from the floor. To do this, your legs have to stay down. However, because your legs are lighter than your trunk, the tendency is for the legs to lift, unless the trunk is bent. Bending the trunk reduces the effect of leverage, and makes the trunk 'lighter'.

As an example of this mechanism, study fig. 6.1. Two boys are sitting on a seesaw. The one on the right weighs 22 kg (50 lb), but the boy on the left is heavier and weighs 27 kg (60 lb). The seesaw is balanced at the moment, but if the lighter boy wants to lift the heavier boy, the heavier boy must move closer to the pivot point. This reduces his leverage effect and can be thought of as making him 'lighter'.

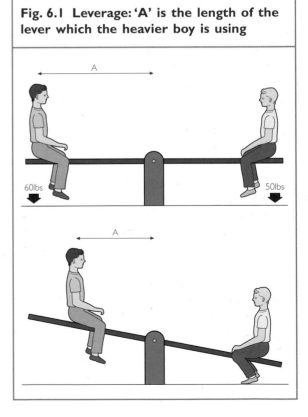

Fig. 6.1 Leverage: 'A' is the length of the lever which the heavier boy is using

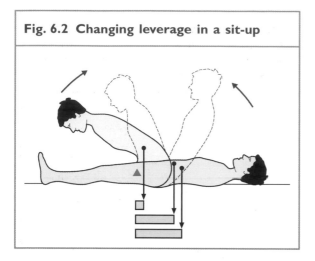

Fig. 6.2 Changing leverage in a sit-up

Fig. 6.3 (a) when the hip flexors pull they can arch the spine; (b) bending the knees reduces spinal compression; (c) in the lying position the hip flexors pull parallel to the spine causing little lifting effect but maximal spinal compression

a.

hip flexor muscle

b.

direction of muscle pull

c.

The same principle applies with the sit-up. If the trunk is to lift instead of the legs, the leverage effect of the trunk must be reduced. To do this the trunk must bend so that its weight moves closer to the hip which is acting as the pivot (*see* fig. 6.2). If you are able to bend your trunk sufficiently, you will be able to sit up. But, if your abdominal muscles are weak or lengthened, your trunk will not bend enough to reduce its leverage; your trunk will stay on the ground and your legs will lift instead.

The abdominal muscles work to bend the trunk, but the lifting action which pulls the trunk away from the floor is actually carried out by the hip flexor muscles. The two major hip flexor muscles are the iliopsoas which attaches to the pelvis and lumbar spine and the rectus femoris which attaches to the pelvis.

> ### Keypoint
>
> The two major hip flexor muscles are the iliopsoas and rectus femoris.

These will pull hard on the spine to try to lift it up. If the legs are straight, the hip flexor muscles lie almost parallel to the spine (*see* fig. 6.3c). The muscles find it very difficult to lift the spine from this position, and instead they pull the lower spine into an arched position (*see* fig. 6.3a).

Bending the knees

If the knees and hips are bent (*see* fig. 6.3b), the hip flexor muscles are lifted up and they can now move the spine more easily and, as a result, will compress it less. Bending the hip therefore considerably reduces the stress placed on the lumbar spine.

Bending the knees protects the spine from muscle compression, but it does have a downside. With the knees bent, the hip flexor muscles can work harder and are in a shortened position. In people who have a hollow back (lordotic) posture these muscles tend to be too tight and too short. To tighten and shorten the muscles further will degrade their posture and could increase the risk of developing back pain.

It must be emphasised that the stress on the spine from hip flexor action only occurs because the trunk is lifted clear of the ground. The action of lifting the trunk rather than simply curling it does not increase the work of the abdominals substantially, and is really unnecessary in pure abdominal training. If the trunk stays on the ground, with the abdominals being used to bend the trunk only, the effects on the lumbar spine are reduced once again and the exercise becomes quite safe.

Fixing the feet

Fixing the feet during a sit-up enables you to pull harder with the hip flexor muscles. This in turn can increase the stress on the spine, and allow you to sit up without needing to bend your spine. The effect is therefore to increase the work of the hip flexors but reduce the work of the abdominals, precisely the opposite to what we require from the exercise. In this programme we do not use foot fixation for basic abdominal exercises.

Inclining the sit-up bench changes the leverage effect on the spine (*see* fig. 6.4). In a normal sit-up (*see* fig. 6.4a) performed from the

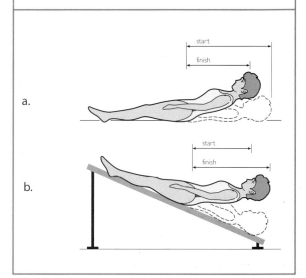

Fig. 6.4 The inclined sit-up: (a) leverage reduces as movement continues; (b) leverage increases up to the mid-point of the movement

floor, the leverage acting on the trunk is maximum at the beginning of the exercise. As the trunk lifts, the leverage reduces. If we incline the sit-up bench, however (*see* fig. 6.4b), the leverage lessens at the beginning of the movement but increases to its maximum about halfway through the exercise as the body moves into the horizontal position. As the trunk lifts further, it moves away from the horizontal and so the leverage forces reduce again. Inclining the bench therefore makes the exercise harder.

The leg raise

The leg raise can in some ways be seen as the reverse of the sit-up. With this exercise, the trunk stays on the ground and the legs are lifted instead. The movement now is purely from the hip flexors; they work to pull the legs up from the ground. However, again because the hip flexor muscles lie parallel with the spine, they will tend to arch the lumbar spine and subject it to forces large enough to damage it severely. The problem occurs because as well as attaching to the lumbar spine, the hip flexors attach to the pelvis. As they pull, they tend to tip the pelvis and pull the lumbar spine out of alignment. Normally the abdominal muscles will contract to stop this unwanted action occurring (*see* fig. 6.5a). If they are weak, however, the abdominals will be unable to do this and the pelvis will tilt, placing stress on the lumbar spine (*see* fig. 6.5b).

The problem can be greatly reduced if the legs are bent to reduce their leverage effect (*see* fig. 6.5c). The reduced leverage means that the abdominal muscles do not have to work as hard to hold the pelvis and lumbar spine in place. If they are weak, the abdominals may only be able to hold the pelvis still against the reduced leverage of the bent legs. In addition, if the hips are bent, the hip flexors can now pull at an angle rather than parallel to the spine. They will therefore compress the spine less and become more effective in creating hip movement instead.

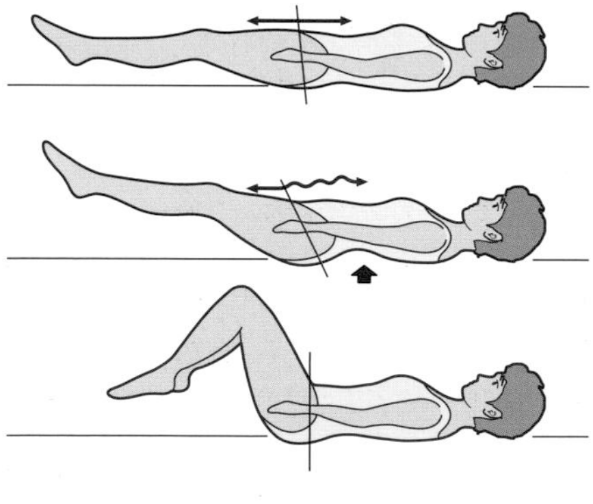

Leverage forces applied from the legs are greatest when the leg is horizontal. If you choose to perform this exercise, make sure you keep the legs away from the horizontal. This can be achieved by performing the exercise against a wall with the legs beginning vertical. As the legs lower, the pelvis must be kept still. If it begins to tip, the exercise should stop because the abdominal muscles are failing to hold the pelvis stable. At this point, the legs are rested against the wall to take the weight off the spine. The movement is now to lower the legs from the vertical towards the wall rather than raising them from the floor.

The same reservation applies with this exercise as with the sit-up. The hip flexors are working primarily, and the abdominals are holding the spine still. If we want to work the abdominals harder, we must modify the leg raise so that the spine bends and the tail lifts off the ground. This exercise is the pelvic raise, sometimes called the reverse crunch. It is described on page 121.

Fig. 6.5 The leg raise: (a) as the hip flexor muscles pull on the pelvis, the abdominals stop the pelvis from tilting; (b) if the abdominals are weak, the pelvis tips forward, hollowing the lower back as the legs are lifted; (c) bending the knees reduces the leverage effect

a.

b.

c.

Keypoint

Do not allow the legs to move into a horizontal position when performing a leg raise.

The trunk crunch

The trunk crunch is a modification of the standard sit-up originally used by professional bodybuilders. It is an intense exercise and not suitable for the novice.

The exercise begins lying on the floor on your back. The knees and hips are bent to 90 degrees, and the calves are placed on a bench or chair. From this position a sit-up is performed, moving the head towards the knees.

The exercise begins in the same way as the sit-up, with the abdominal muscles working hard. Because the pelvis remains still, the emphasis of the exercise is on the upper abdominals with the lower portion of the muscles showing less activity. As the spine bends maximally you reach a point where you must lift yourself up from the floor. In lighter subjects this may not be possible, but those who have heavier legs will be able to achieve this movement. Performing the action with the legs fixed enables you to pull the feet against the fixation point. As this happens the hip flexor muscles pull hard to lift the spine off the ground.

If the action is performed with a twist, the oblique abdominals will work more, but the central abdominal muscle (rectus abdominis) will still work hard.

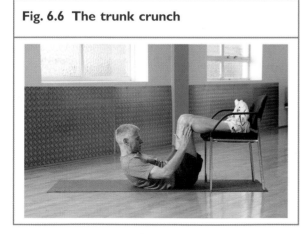

Fig. 6.6 The trunk crunch

Although a useful exercise because it strongly emphasises the upper portion of the abdominal muscles, the trunk crunch must be balanced out by using the pelvic raise to work the lower portion of the muscles. Failure to do this will leave an imbalance between the upper and lower portion of the abdominals, a situation which could lead to back pain.

> ### Keypoint
>
> The trunk crunch is an advanced exercise to be used only after initial abdominal strength has been gained using other exercises. The crunch focuses on the upper abdominal region, and must be balanced by movements which emphasise the lower abdominal area, such as the pelvic raise.

The trunk crunch is not suitable for those who have suffered from persistent back pain or who require light training. It is included as an advanced exercise in this book performed with the feet free (not fixed) initially to reduce stress on the lower spine.

The knee raise (hip flexor)

The hip flexor station is a standard machine in many gyms and is often seen as an attachment to multi-station weight training units. The machine consists of a back pad and two side gutter pads to take the forearms.

Normal instructions are to lift yourself up into the machine with your elbows bent to 90 degrees and your forearms in the gutter pads (*see* fig. 6.7). The small of your back is pressed against the back pad. From this position lift your legs, keeping them straight, to the horizontal position and then lower them down again.

As the legs lift, the hip flexors work. To stabilise the spine and pelvis the abdominal muscles tighten. Only when the spine begins to bend, as the legs near the horizontal position, do the abdominals work to actually bend the spine. Although the exercise feels hard, the greatest amount of the work is from the hip flexors, with the abdominals receiving only a poor workout.

One of the major problems with this exercise stems from the length of the hamstring muscles on the back of the thigh. In many people these muscles are very short. When this is the case, you are not able to lift the legs out straight without the knees bending. If you try to hold the knees straight, the tight hamstrings will pull on the pelvis and cause the lower spine to bend. This can place stress on the spine.

A second area of concern is due to momentum. Because some people find the exercise hard, there is a tendency to swing the legs to assist the movement. When this happens, the momentum of the heavy legs moving at speed becomes uncontrollable. As the legs are lowered, they swing backwards forcing the back to hyperextend (*see* fig. 6.6b) and severely stressing the spine.

The hip flexor exercise can be made safer and more effective with some modifications. Firstly, the knees should be bent to relax the hamstrings and so reduce the stress on the lower back. In addition, bending the knees reduces the leverage effect and makes the exercise more controllable. If the knees are bent to 90 degrees and kept still, the action can then be one of bending the trunk to pull the tailbone away from the pad (*see* fig. 6.6c). This increases the emphasis on the abdominal muscles, making the exercise more effective. Secondly, any swinging of the legs should be avoided. As the legs are lowered they should be under control. In the bottom position, pause before you start to lift the legs again. In this way momentum is cut down and the back is not forced into an unnatural position.

Fig. 6.7 The knee raise: (a) the abdominals work to hold the pelvis firm at the beginning of the movement; (b) if the legs are allowed to swing backwards, the lower back will hollow dangerously (hyper-extend); (c) knees and hips bent to 90 degrees; (d) trunk flexes to lift legs

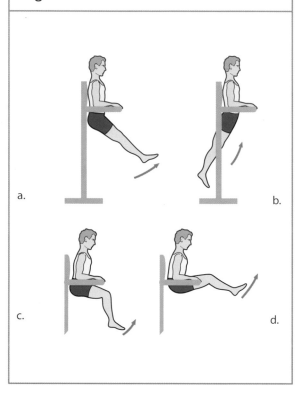

Keypoint

The knee raise can place stress on the lower back if it is performed with a 'swinging' action. Keep the action under control at all times, especially when lowering the legs.

TRUNK EXERCISE DANGERS

7

More than any other area in the body, the back is susceptible to injury through incorrect exercise. To prevent injury, we need to have an understanding of some basic mechanical concepts.

Leverage

The limbs and spine act as levers when we move. A lever is simply a rigid bar which moves around a fixed point or pivot. Two forces act on the lever: effort and resistance. The effort tries to move the lever, while the resistance tries to stop movement. In the body, the effort is supplied by your muscles, while the resistance is the weight of the moving body part. Take as an example the leg lifting from a lying position. The pivot is the hip joint, the effort is supplied by the hip flexor muscles which lift the leg, and the resistance is the weight of the whole leg. The effort from the muscle acts at the point where the muscle attaches to the thighbone (*see* fig. 7.1b).

We say that the weight acts through a single point called the 'centre of gravity'. This is really the balance point of the limb, and would be the centre point of the limb if the limb were the same size all over. However, because the leg is thicker at the top, the centre of gravity lies towards the heavier end.

> ### Keypoint
> The centre of gravity of a limb is its balance point.

Leverage is greater when there is a long horizontal distance between the pivot and the

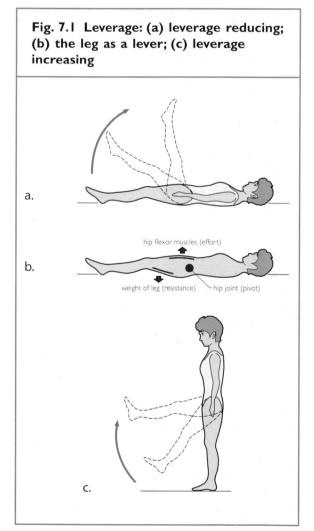

Fig. 7.1 Leverage: (a) leverage reducing; (b) the leg as a lever; (c) leverage increasing

a.

b. hip flexor muscles (effort)

weight of leg (resistance)   hip joint (pivot)

c.

point where the weight or effort acts. In fig. 7.1, the leverage is greatest when the leg first lifts from the ground, because it is close to the horizontal. As the leg lifts up, it moves away from the horizontal and so the leverage reduces and the exercise actually gets easier. In fig. 7.1c the subject is standing up with the legs in the vertical position. The leverage to begin with is minimal. As the leg lifts, however, it moves towards the horizontal and so the leverage increases. This is now the reverse situation to fig. 7.1a, and the exercise gradually gets harder. Although both exercises involve flexing the straight leg, the starting position of the movement changes the effect of the exercise considerably.

Keypoint

Leverage is greatest when a lever is in a horizontal position.

This example has important implications with regards to the safety of the spine. Exercises which involve moving the spine into a horizontal position will place great amounts of leverage on the spine and should be used with caution. Often, simply altering the starting position will move the spine away from the horizontal and so reduce the stress on the lower back. Where a horizontal position must be used, the spine should be supported. As an example of this process let's look at a common stretch for the hamstring muscles on the back of the thigh. In fig. 7.2a an athlete is stretching the hamstrings by bending the trunk forwards from the hip. This action places an excessive leverage stress on the spine because it is moving from a vertical position (minimal leverage) to a more horizontal position (maximum leverage). Simply by placing one hand down on the knee, the spine is supported and the stress reduced (*see* fig. 7.2b).

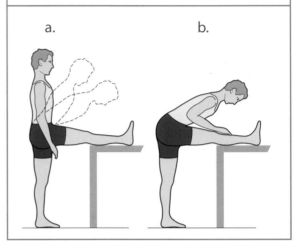

Fig. 7.2 Supporting the body when leverage is large: (a) spine moves towards the horizontal, leverage increases; (b) bodyweight taken through the arm at the point of maximum leverage

a.   b.

Keypoint

If an exercise doesn't allow you to keep your spine vertical, place your hand on something for support.

Which body area is moving?

Often, a quick look at an exercise creates the impression that a particular part of the body is moving. On closer inspection, however, it can be seen that other body areas are also moving and these may be taking greater stress than is intended. This holds true particularly with the pelvis moving on the spine or hip. Take as an example a stretch for the thigh muscles (*see* fig. 7.3). The subject is standing up straight and has grasped the ankle. She is pulling the hip backwards and trying to increase the bend on the knee at the same time. At first sight this seems

Fig. 7.3 (a) Normal pelvic tilt and lower back alignment; (b) pelvis moves excessively, causing lower back to hollow: leg goes higher, but technique is faulty

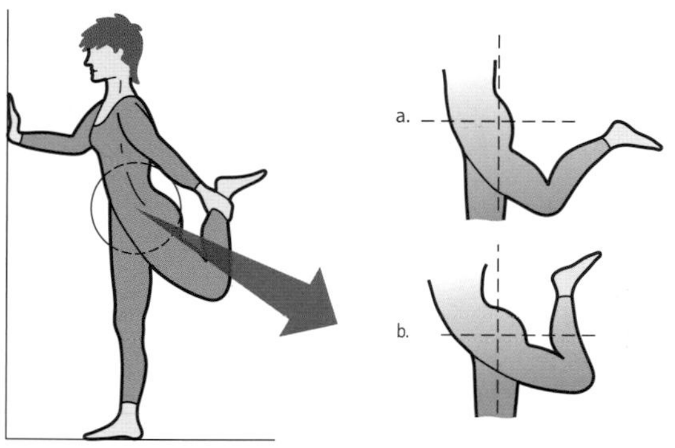

Fig. 7.4 (a) Normal movement; (b) excessive movement of upper spine

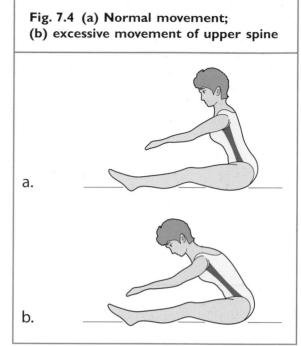

to be an exercise which is simply placing the thigh muscles into a stretch. However, if we look closely we can see that the pelvis has tilted forwards and stress is now placed on the spine. In this case the spine is more flexible than the tight thigh muscles, so the more the stretch is pushed, the more stress is thrown onto the spine.

If we look at fig. 7.4, the subject is trying to touch her toes by stretching her hamstrings (behind the thigh). In fig. 7.4b she appears to be stretching further because she has reached closer to her toes. However, if we look at the line of the pelvis, the subject has moved exactly the same amount both times. The extra movement in fig. 7.4b has occurred by over-bending the upper spine. Again, this part of the body is generally more flexible than the tight hamstrings. As the movement is pushed further and further, the stretch on the hamstrings will not increase, but the stress on the upper spine certainly will.

Keypoint

Looking at the pelvis gives an important indication of lumbar spine position.

Momentum

Momentum is a combination of how heavy an object is and how quickly it is moving. A heavy object, such as the leg or trunk, which is moving quickly, will possess a great deal of momentum and will be very difficult to stop. The high momentum can take over the movement, and you may find that you are no longer able to control a body part. This is when injuries can occur.

There are two methods to make this type of exercise safer. Firstly, you can reduce the momentum by slowing the movement down where heavy body parts are used. In this book all movements of the trunk are slow to begin with. It is only when we have a considerable degree of control over an action that the speed is increased.

The second way to make a movement safer, if it is moving quickly, is to ensure that the movement only occurs in the middle of the joint range. The joint range is the total movement from one extreme to the other. In the case of the knee, it would be from the fully bent position to fully straight. Where an action is rapid, we must restrict the movement to the middle part of this range so that the joint is never fully bent or fully straightened. In this way we reduce the likelihood of injuring the joint tissues by overstretching them.

Keypoint

Keep movements slow and controlled. Use the middle of a joint's total movement more often than the ends.

Excessive lumbar curvature

We have seen earlier that pelvic tilt is intimately linked with lumbar curvature. Tilting the pelvis forwards increases the lumbar curve, while tilting it backwards flattens it. One of the aims of the foundation movements in this book (chapter 9) is to enable a subject to identify the neutral position of the spine, where the pelvis is level, and to hold this position while performing other movements. This control is an important component of core stability and lays the foundation of good abdominal training. Only when core stability is good should someone progress to harder exercise.

If the pelvis is allowed to tilt too far, the lumbar spine will move to its end point. At this point the disc, spinal facet joints and lumbar tissues are all stressed excessively. Increasing the curve will press the facet joints together, while flattening the curve will push the spinal disc backwards. In each case, the ligaments surrounding the spinal tissues are overstretched.

A number of abdominal exercises will tend to increase the lumbar curve dangerously. In the straight leg raise action (*see* fig. 7.5a), the pull of the hip muscles on to the pelvis and lumbar spine tends to tilt the pelvis forwards and lift the lumbar spine away from the ground. Even if the spine remains flat on the floor, the hip muscles still pull dangerously hard on to the lower spine, compressing the discs and increasing the likelihood of injury. The safer alternative to this exercise is the heel slide (*see* page 103). Now only one leg is lifting at a time, the other one remaining on the floor to provide support and increase stability. In addition, the heel of the leg which moves stays on the ground so the full weight is not lifted.

With spinal hyperextension exercises in an unsupported position (*see* fig. 7.5b), the abdominal muscles may be unable to support the spine and hold it in its neutral position. As a consequence, the pelvis tilts forwards and the lumbar spine moves too far into extension. As we have seen, this position compresses the joints in the base of the spine. This compression is compounded by the powerful contraction of the spinal extensor muscles which are fighting to hold the body up. Alternatives to this exercise include bridging (exercise 44, page 125) and the spinal extension hold (exercise 72, page 157). In each case the whole bodyweight is not taken until all the trunk muscles are strong enough to do this. When the muscles are strong, the pelvis is aligned and the abdominal hollowing procedure is practised first, before the exercise begins. In this way the spine is correctly aligned before it is loaded.

Overhead pressing actions in weight training can also lead to hyperextension of the lumbar spine through the pelvis tilt mechanism if the abdominal muscles fail to contract at the onset of the lift (*see* fig. 7.5c). To prevent this happening, firstly the abdominal hollowing procedure must be practised throughout the lift. Secondly, the limiting factor should not be the amount of weight that can be lifted overhead, but the point at which the pelvis begins to tilt. When this happens, the exercise must stop, however large or small the weight being lifted.

Flattening of the lumbar spine is common in sitting positions. Squatting on to a bench which is too low, for example (*see* fig. 7.5d), will allow the pelvis to tilt backwards and this in turn pulls the spinal bones into a flexed position. Done at speed, this type of action can be extremely dangerous. The movement can be modified in two ways. Firstly, the bench height must be adjusted so that it is just higher than the subject's knee. In this way the amount of knee and hip movement is reduced and the lumbar spine will not be rounded as far. Secondly, the movement should be slowed down so that the momentum is reduced. In this way, less stress is passed on to the spine, and the action stays controlled all the time.

> **Keypoint**
>
> Try to keep your spine in the neutral position as often as possible.

Neck posture

In an earlier section we saw that the posture line can be used to determine optimal posture. With reference to the head and neck, the posture line should pass through the shoulder joint and also through the ear. A common faulty

Fig. 7.5 Excessive lumbar curvature

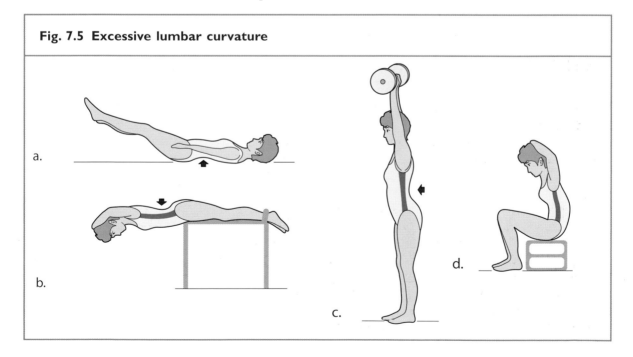

a.

b.

c.

d.

alignment seen in exercise is where the head is held forward (*see* fig. 7.6). The ear can be seen to move about 5–10 cm (2–4 inches) forwards of the posture line and well in front of the shoulder. This stresses the neck tissues and is very dangerous when performed at speed. The movement is common when the head is used to lead, and provides momentum to get an action started. This is especially true of sit-up-type exercises. If a subject is attempting to sit up from the ground, they may be unable to do so if their abdominal muscles are very weak. One way that they can cover this up is to perform the action quickly and use the weight of the head to 'fling' the body off the ground. This rapid action can damage the neck structures sufficiently to cause a trapped nerve and even a type of whiplash injury.

To avoid this neck posture, the chin should be held back, in alignment with the rest of the spine. This position is held so the head does not move, and the action is performed slowly, under control.

During a trunk curl action, the chin should be held in slightly, so that the neck muscles are active to support the upper spine. A good teaching point to keep the chin tucked in is to

Keypoint

Avoid nodding your head when performing abdominal exercises.

grip a tennis ball lightly under the chin. This gives just the right amount of chin tuck without bending (flexing) the neck too far.

Forcing the neck into end range postures is also a cause for concern. Placing the hands behind the neck and pulling hard when performing any curling action can dangerously stress the tissues of the upper spine (*see* fig. 7.7). This not only stresses the muscles and ligaments, but can cut off the blood flow travelling through the neck to the head, and stretch the brain stem (the connection between the spine and brain) itself. This can cause a person to get dizzy and even pass out in some cases. Only use the hands behind the neck to take the weight of the head, and rest the head lightly in the hands. Do not force the neck into flexion.

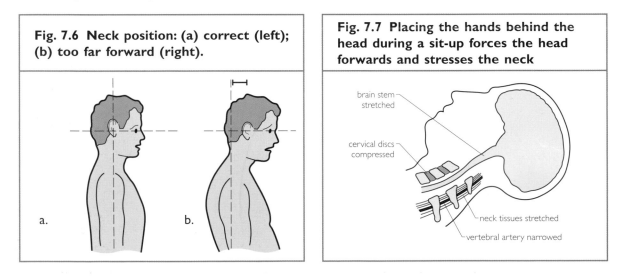

Fig. 7.6 Neck position: (a) correct (left); (b) too far forward (right).

a.   b.

Fig. 7.7 Placing the hands behind the head during a sit-up forces the head forwards and stresses the neck

brain stem stretched

cervical discs compressed

neck tissues stretched

vertebral artery narrowed

Stability

Three factors are important to stability: the size and alignment of the base of support, and the centre of gravity. An object's base of support is the total area that is on the ground or, in the case of the human body, the distance between the feet (*see* fig. 7.8). If the base of support is wide, the weight of the object is distributed over a large area and the object is therefore stable, like a pyramid. When the base of support is small, as with a ballet dancer *en point*, the object is unstable and likely to wobble off balance. When choosing an exercise position, therefore, we should make sure that our base of support is as wide as is comfortable.

The second factor concerning the base of support which is important to stability is the direction in which it faces. Aligning your feet so that they face the way you are moving makes you more stable. For example, if you have your feet one in front of the other, although your base of support is large, you will still be unstable if you are practising a side bend movement. This is because the side bend movement occurs in a side-to-side direction, but your feet position has widened your base of support in a forward-to-back direction. To be stable while performing side bends, your feet must be apart in a sideways direction. Similarly, if your feet are apart sideways you are unstable when performing shoulder rounding and bracing. This movement occurs front-to-back, so your base of support should be widened in this direction.

The third factor which is important to stability is the height of your bodyweight above the ground. When you stand tall, you are less stable and there is a tendency to topple when performing exercises. Simply bending your knees lowers your bodyweight closer to the ground and makes you more stable.

Fig. 7.8 Stability: grey area is the base of support (a) stable when wide; (b) unstable – small base of support; (c) base is wide in direction of movement – stable; (d) base is widened in direction different to movement – less stable

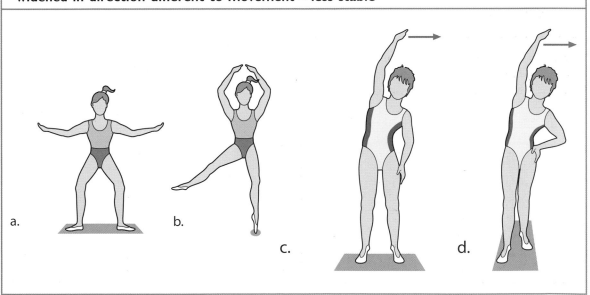

a.   b.   c.   d.

Comfort

An exercise which is uncomfortable can also be dangerous. When you are not comfortable you tend to alter your posture regularly, and wriggle. This takes concentration away from the exercise and affects stability. An exercise usually becomes uncomfortable if you are placing weight through a bony point such as the knee, hip or tailbone, and pressure builds up. In each of these cases try to rest the body part on a mat or folded towel instead of on the floor alone.

Taking up an unnatural posture will also make you uncomfortable as it will stress the body tissues excessively. When using equipment, therefore, make sure it is adjusted to suit your body size. This is especially true of weight training apparatus where correct seat height adjustment is vital to allow correct spinal alignment.

Summary

- The centre of gravity of an object is its balance point.
- In a lever, the further away from the pivot a weight is placed, the greater the leverage effect.
- Momentum is a combination of how heavy an object is and how fast it is moving.
- Tilting the pelvis *forwards increases* the lumbar curve; tilting *backwards decreases* it.
- Maintain good alignment of your neck when exercising. Don't allow your chin to poke forwards, or pull hard on your neck.
- Stability is determined by the size and alignment of an object's base of support and the position of its centre of gravity.

BEFORE WE START

8

Warm-up

Before starting an abdominal training session, it is vital to warm up. There are two main reasons for this: first, warming up can make sports injuries less likely in certain circumstances, and this is especially true for the spine; second, the body works more efficiently when warm and body functions may actually improve. A good warm-up will have effects in three key areas: physiological (body processes), mechanical (physics of body tissues) and psychological (the mind).

Physiological effects

It takes some time for the body to change from its basic 'tick over' at rest to a point at which it is ready to perform maximally. If vigorous exercise is started immediately from rest, the heartbeat is speeded up with a sudden jolt instead of increasing gradually, and the beats of the heart can become irregular (*ectopic beats*), rather than showing their normal smooth rhythm. These changes affecting the heart can be potentially very serious in the older or less active individual, and especially in those with a history of heart or circulatory problems.

Effects on the heart

Over 40 years ago a research study was conducted which clearly illustrated the effects of a warm-up on the heart. Researchers took a group of men with no history of heart problems and made them run vigorously on a treadmill for 10–15 seconds without a warm-up. In 70 per cent of these subjects, abnormal changes were seen on an electrocardiogram (ECG) machine. These changes, called *ischaemia*, showed that insufficient blood was getting to the heart muscle, a potentially very dangerous situation. However, when the same subjects ran on the treadmill after performing a warm-up, the ECG changes were greatly reduced, and in many cases the heartbeat was completely normal. In addition, blood pressure (BP) was taken when the subjects ran on the treadmill both with and without a warm-up. Blood pressure for those who used a warm-up was on average 12 per cent lower than those who did not.

Effect on body tissue

A warm-up will allow the body tissues to work more efficiently. Normally, while relaxed, the muscles receive only about 15 per cent of the total blood flow. The rest of the blood goes to the body organs such as the brain, liver and intestines. During vigorous exercise, because the muscles need far more fuel to provide energy, their requirement for blood increases to 80 per cent of the total blood flow. It takes time to re-route this blood by opening some blood vessels and closing others, and if the muscles are required to perform maximally before the blood flow has changed they will work inefficiently.

Lactic acid formation

The body can produce energy by two methods: aerobically (with oxygen) and anaerobically (without oxygen). The aerobic method is preferable, because when we work anaerobically we produce a waste product called *lactic acid.* Unfortunately, we cannot work aerobically straightaway as it takes time to switch the aerobic system on. If we start intense exercise without a warm-up, the aerobic system does not have enough time to switch on; we therefore have to provide energy anaerobically, with resultant lactic acid formation.

The function of a warm-up is to 'switch on' the aerobic system and allow the body to reach a steady state where the energy provided by the body exactly matches its requirements through exercise. Once this is done, less waste is produced and so our recovery after exercise will be much faster.

Mechanical effect

The mechanical effects of warm-up occur as a direct result of tissue heating. Chemical reactions involved in the production of energy for the working muscle and the removal of waste products are speeded up with warmth. In addition, nerve impulses travel faster when a nerve is warm. The effects of a warm-up on nerve conduction is particularly important for the speed of reflexes, which protect the muscles from injury, an essential component of core stability.

When a substance is heated it becomes more pliable, and this is exactly the same for the body tissues and the fluids within joints. Fluids are fairly stiff (viscous) at rest but become thinner and more malleable with movement. The facet joints of the spine contain fluid, as do the discs, so the spine is affected by this change in viscosity. The overall effect of a warm-up on the spine is to make it less stiff and so make movements smoother and easier to control.

Psychological effects

Two effects are important here: *arousal level* and *mental rehearsal.*

Arousal level

Arousal level is how alert you are. There is a direct relationship between arousal and performance. Initially, as arousal increases so does performance. However, after a certain point an individual becomes too aroused (they are now 'stressed') and their performance suffers. As an illustration of this mechanism, imagine you have had a boring day and you arrive at the gym not really wanting to exercise. Your arousal level is low so your exercise performance will be poor. If you then go into an exercise class, however, the instructor, the music and the other people, will increase your arousal level. You feel motivated and your exercise performance improves.

Now imagine if you are an athlete competing in an important game and you miss a shot that normally you would find very easy. Perhaps you are nervous, your heart is pounding and your arousal level is too high, so your performance suffers.

The function of a warm-up should be to make someone optimally aroused. Not too little so they are not alert, and not too much so they are stressed.

> ## Keypoint
>
> A good warm-up will make a person optimally aroused for sport. An anxious individual is calmed down and an under-motivated individual is 'psyched up'.

Mental rehearsal

The second psychological effect of a warm-up is mental rehearsal. Complex actions tend to be forgotten between exercise bouts – and remember that many of the movements used in core stability can seem complex when you first use them. The first or second repetition of a complex action may not be as good as the fourth or fifth, when you have had time to 'get into' the movement. With skilled actions such as lifting and twisting it is essential that we rehearse the movement, slowly going through the movement before we perform the action at full speed. Uncoordinated actions on the spine are a recipe for injury.

Types of warm-up

A warm-up can either be *passive* with the body heated from the outside, or *active*, using exercise to form the heat internally. An example of a passive warm-up is to have a sauna or hot shower. An active warm-up can be achieved through gentle jogging or using light aerobics. Both types can be effective, but are appropriate in different situations.

An active warm-up is the type normally used before exercise, while the passive warm-up is useful when stretching a muscle tightened from a previous strain, for example. The advantage of the passive warm-up, from the point of view of injury, is that it does not require the user to move the injured tissues in order to create body heat. The use of external heat can also reduce pain and muscle spasm, helping tissues to relax and allowing them to move more comfortably.

In addition to active and passive types, a warm-up may also be either *general* or *specific*. A general warm-up, such as jogging or static cycling, will affect the whole body. The effects here are mainly on the major body systems such as the heart, lungs and blood vessels. This should be followed by a specific warm-up which concentrates on the body part and action to be used in a particular exercise. The effects now are more localised, mainly targeting the body tissues used in the actual exercise and rehearsing the action to be performed.

Warm-up techniques

Clothing for a warm-up should enable you to maintain body heat and allow unrestricted movement. Shorts and a T-shirt are fine for warmer weather, but fleecy jogging bottoms and a sweatshirt are normally better when it is cooler. Remember that you may need to see your spine in the mirror at some stage of the exercise programme, so try to wear layers of clothing which you can gradually remove.

Make sure that you can move without restriction from furniture or other people. A little time spent clearing some space in the room you are using is worthwhile. You may

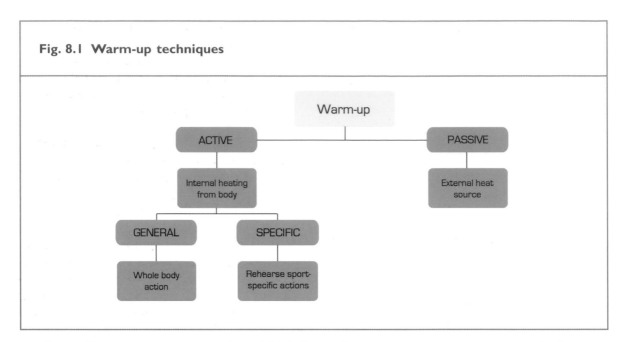

Fig. 8.1 Warm-up techniques

need a small exercise mat or a number of folded towels at hand for padding during exercises where you are kneeling or lying on the floor.

The amount of exercise required for an effective warm-up will depend very much on a person's fitness level and the exercise to be performed in the main part of the workout. This is because changes in body temperature vary with body size, fat level and rate of body metabolism. In addition, activities differ tremendously in the demand they make on the body tissues, so a warm-up before a vigorous game of hockey, for example, would need to be more extensive than one for a casual game of bowls.

Here are some guidelines before we get onto warm-up prior to abdominal exercise.

- **Intensity**: If it is to be effective, a warm-up must be intense enough to cause mild sweating. This has been shown to be the minimum intensity to bring about the warm-up changes discussed above.
- **Clothing**: Because we are trying to raise the body temperature, it is best to perform

the warm-up wearing warm clothing to keep the body heat in.
- **Activities**: Warm-up activities should be continuous and rhythmical in nature. Gentle jogging, light aerobics, or cycling on a static bicycle in the gym are all examples of good warm-up activities. Aim to sweat lightly, take the major joints through their full range of movement and, finally, to perform some sport-specific actions as a part of skill rehearsal.
- **Time**: A good warm-up may take 10–15 minutes if it is before intense competitive actions, 2–3 minutes before less intense movement.

Keypoint

Match your warm-up to your body requirements and the exercise type and intensity.

Example warm-up for abdominal training

Divide the warm-up into three sections: firstly the *pulse raiser*, secondly *mobility* and thirdly *movement rehearsal.*

The pulse raising activity may be a brisk walk (wear well-padded shoes to minimise jarring) or a cycle on a static bike in the gym, for example. Perform 2–5 minutes so that you feel warm and begin to sweat lightly. Then, move onto the mobility exercises:

• **Shoulders**: hold on to a towel and simply reach overhead, keeping the arms straight. Do not arch the back while doing this, and make sure that the movement is slow and controlled.
• **Spinal twist**: slowly turn so that you look to the right and then to the left, gently twisting the whole of the spine, including the neck, thoracic spine (chest level) and lumbar spine (lower back).
• **Side bending**: rest the hands slightly below the hips, at mid-thigh level. Use the hands for support and slowly bend to the right and then stand straight again. Repeat the action to the left.
• **Hip mobility**: hold on to the back of a chair and raise one knee as far as you can towards the chest, bending at both the knee and the hip. Make sure you keep standing straight and do not bend your spine.

Finally, rehearse two important exercises from the foundation section (chapter 9): abdominal hollowing to remind yourself how to work the core stability muscles and the pelvic tilt to rehearse subtle control of the lumbar (low back) curve.

Table 8.1	Example warm-up	
Aim	**Action**
• Raise pulse rate	• Static cycle or brisk walking in well-padded shoes – 2–5 mins
• Mobility of shoulders, hips and spine	• Overhead reach – 10 reps • Flexion-extension of lumbar spine with pelvic tilt (see below) • Rotation of lumbar spine – 5 reps to each side • Side bending of lumbar spine – 5 reps to each side • Knee lifts – 5 reps each knee
• Rehearse foundation actions	• Pelvic tilting, standing (page 87) – 3 reps • Abdominal hollowing, standing (page 94) – 3 reps

Warm-down

Just as it is vital to begin an exercise session slowly by warming up, so it is important to end it the same way by using a warm-down or cool-down. The warm-down period has a number of important effects.

First, during intense exercise the heartbeat increases, and the beating of the heart is actually helped by the contraction of the exercising limb muscles. As these muscles contract they squeeze the blood vessels which travel through them, thus helping the blood to return to the heart – this process is called the *auxiliary muscle pump.* If you stop exercising abruptly, the heart must work harder because the muscle pump has stopped. In this case your pulse will actually get faster although exercise has stopped.

An effective warm-down can also reduce muscle ache. This is caused partly by lactic acid formed as a waste product of muscle contraction, and partly through tiny muscle tears which occur during very hard training. Hard training causes local swelling within a muscle, giving *delayed onset muscle soreness* (DOMS). In the case of DOMS, you feel fine the day after a workout, but the day after that you feel stiff.

To reduce these effects you should perform a warm-down using similar exercises to those chosen for the warm-up, gradually lowering the exercise intensity until resting levels are reached. Finally, shake your muscles to loosen and relax them, and take a warm shower to flush fresh blood through them and aid recovery. Because blood is still needed in the muscles after exercise to aid recovery, you should not eat a large meal immediately. If you feel hungry and in need of an 'energy boost' eat a small amount of sweet, high-carbohydrate food such as a banana or toast and honey.

Keypoint

When planning your workout allow at least 5 minutes for a warm-down.

FOUNDATION

9

We begin abdominal training by establishing core stability and learning precise control of the lumbo-pelvis, the junction between the lower back and the pelvic region. The reason for this foundation is two-fold. Firstly, poorly controlled movements are always risky from the point of view of injuries; poorly controlled movements performed on an unstable spine are almost guaranteed to lead to injury sooner or later. Secondly, by performing abdominal exercise in an imprecise way we are rehearsing poor movement patterns which will be very hard to 'un-learn' later. It's a little like walking before you can run. If you start walking with a limp, by the time you begin running everything will be sore!

Let's start by mastering two essential movements which form the cornerstones of good abdominal training: pelvic tilting and abdominal hollowing.

Pelvic tilting

We saw on page 11 that the tilt of the pelvis determines the position of the lower back. Tilting the pelvis forwards increases the hollow in the small of the back (lumbar extension), while tilting the pelvis backwards flattens the back, reducing the lumbar hollow (lumbar flexion). Pelvic tilting is important because it teaches control of the lumbar spine during exercise. An incorrect pelvic tilt during exercise can lead to excessive movement in the lower spine.

We must be able to identify this happening, by feeling the action taking place, so that we can correct it before an injury occurs.

Some people find this movement difficult because their spine is quite stiff. We saw in chapter 4 that posture affects the curve in the base of the spine and the angle of the pelvis. If someone has a hollow back (lordotic) posture, their pelvis is already in anterior tilt. When they try to practise pelvic tilting exercises they will find it very difficult to tilt the pelvis posteriorly and flatten their back. Similarly, someone with a flatback posture has lost their normal lumbar curve (lordosis). They, in turn, will find it very difficult to increase the lumbar curve by tilting the pelvis forwards. Keep going with the exercise, however, because mobility will increase with practice.

Because accurate control of this action is so vital, we will practise the movement from two different starting positions.

Keypoint

Developing accurate control of pelvic tilt is an essential foundation for good abdominal training.

Ex 10 Pelvic tilting, lying

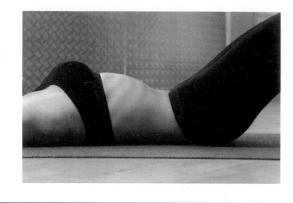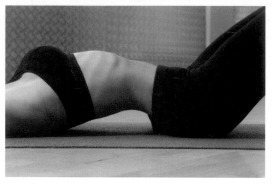

Starting position

Begin lying on your back with your knees bent. Place your feet and knees shoulder-width apart. Your arms should rest on the floor slightly away from your body.

Action

Tighten your abdominal muscles to tip your pelvis backwards, and flatten the small of your back against the floor. Pause and then reverse the action, tightening your back muscles to hollow the small of your back away from the floor. Repeat this action and try to stop the movement when you are halfway between the two extremes. **Note: This mid-point is your neutral position and we will use it later in the programme.**

Points to note

Keeping the knees apart allows the pelvis to move unhindered. If the knees are too close together, free movement of the pelvis will be restricted.

Training tip

The action must be smooth and controlled rather than jerky. A jerking action will stress the lower spine.

Ex 11 Pelvic tilting, standing

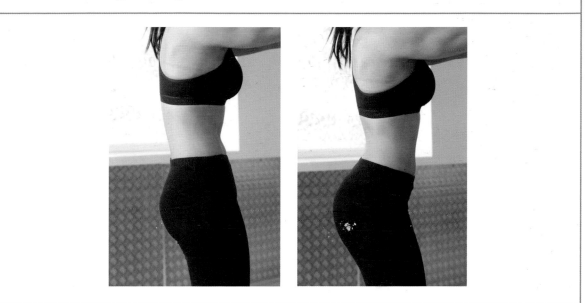

Starting position

Begin standing with your feet shoulder-width apart, arms by your sides. Stand tall. Do not slouch.

Action

Tighten your abdominal muscles and your buttock muscles together to tilt your pelvis backwards and flatten your lower spine. Pause and then tighten your hips and spinal muscles to increase the hollow in the small of your back.

Points to note

The action should be isolated to your lower back. Your shoulders should stay square, and your knees should remain still. Avoid any body sway.

Training tip

Placing your hands out to the side in a 'T' shape will help with the balance of this exercise, and make any unwanted body sway more obvious. If you find it difficult to control body sway, place your hands on a wall in front of you.

Ex 12 Pelvic tilt, bench sitting

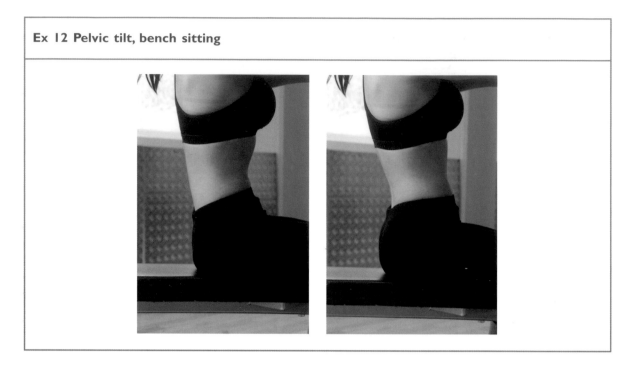

Starting position

Sit on a gym bench or dining chair with your knees bent and slightly apart. Your knees should be positioned slightly lower than your hips. Keep your back straight but not rigid, and your feet flat on the floor.

Action

Sit tall and tilt your pelvis forwards to press your pubic bone towards the bench and hollow your lower back. Pause, and then tilt your pelvis backwards pressing your tailbone (coccyx) onto the bench and flattening your lower back.

Points to note

The movement must be isolated to the pelvis. Do not allow your body to sway and do not round or brace your shoulders.

Training tip

Make sure you keep your knees apart to allow unhindered motion of the pelvis.

Ex 13 Pelvic tilting, on a gym ball

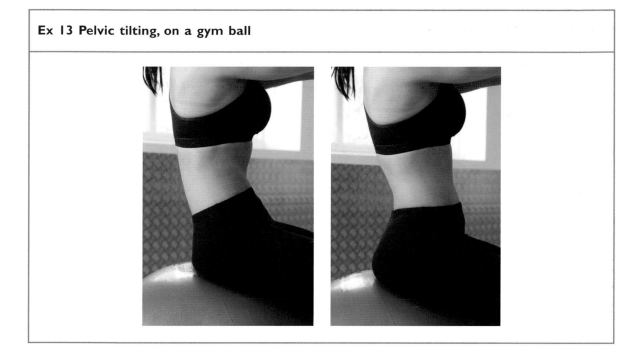

Starting position

Sit on a large 60 cm (24 inch) gym ball with your knees bent to 90 degrees. Your back should be straight but not rigid, and your feet should be flat on the floor.

Action

Sit tall on the ball and tilt your pelvis backwards to decrease the hollow in the small of your back, and then forwards to increase it.

Points to note

The movement must be isolated to the pelvis. Do not allow any body sway and do not round or brace your shoulders.

Training tip

To prevent body sway to begin with, place a dining chair at each side of the ball. Put each hand flat on the chair surfaces to monitor shoulder movement.

Abdominal hollowing

We saw in chapter 2 that the deep abdominal muscles (transversus abdominis and internal oblique) are important muscles to maintain stability of the lower spine. These muscles are often not used in exercise programmes, but it is vital that we work them before we move on to further abdominal training. The muscles work hard during the abdominal hollowing actions described below. Even if you have been training for many years, practise this movement; you may be surprised at just how little control you have in this body area.

General principles with abdominal hollowing

It is important to get the deep corset muscles working. However, sometimes this can be very difficult if the muscles have not worked for a long time or have been damaged. If you have not exercised for a long time, have recently given birth, or had abdominal surgery, this section is especially important for you. Also spend some time reading chapters 14 and 16.

• Starting position

The position that you chose to start your training is important. If you have had back pain, kneeling positions will probably be more comfortable for you. However, if you are very overweight, standing positions are better, because your abdominal muscle movement is more noticeable (and so easier to learn). Sitting and standing positions are both easy to use throughout the day and so are most suitable for home exercise and building your exercise into your daily activities.

• Linking the muscles with pelvic floor contraction

We have seen that the spine is supported by the abdominal balloon mechanism (intra-abdominal pressure). This mechanism involves three components: (i) the abdominal muscles which form the sides of the balloon; (ii) the pelvic floor which forms the floor; and (iii) the diaphragm (sheet of muscle below your chest cavity) which forms the roof. Involving both the pelvic floor and breathing (using the diaphragm) will improve stability and make abdominal exercise both easier to learn and more effective. Look at exercises 12 and 13 pages 88–9, and read the section on the pelvic floor in chapter 14 for more information.

• Breathing

As well as using the diaphragm in abdominal training, you must also make sure that you breath normally and *do not hold your breath* as you practise the exercises. As you contract (tighten) the abdominal muscles try to breathe out.

• Contour of the abdominal wall

As you perform any abdominal exercise the abdominal wall (tummy contour) should stay flat or drawn in slightly (hollow). This action is caused by contraction of the deep muscles (transversus and internal oblique) which 'set' the abdomen before the more powerful surface muscles (rectus and external oblique) come into play. If the deep abdominal muscles do not set the abdomen, the foundation of the movement is lost and you will notice your abdomen bulging or ballooning. This is the time to stop and practise abdominal hollowing actions again before moving on to more general abdominal training.

Ex 14 Abdominal hollowing, kneeling

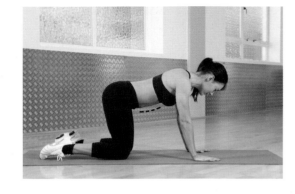 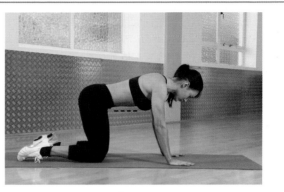

Starting position

Begin kneeling on all fours with your hands and knees shoulder-width apart. Kneel on a mat or folded towel for comfort.

Action

Allow your tummy muscles to relax and sag downwards to the floor. Then tighten them and pull them up and in, trying to hollow your tummy and pull your tummy button (umbilicus) in towards the spine.

Points to note

Initially the amount of movement may be very small, but with practice you should notice 10–15 cm (4–6 inches) of movement in total. Breathe normally throughout the action; do not take a deep breath when trying to flatten your tummy. Keep your spine still as you hollow. Do not arch the spine or tilt the pelvis.

Training tip

(i) Make sure you keep a true 'box' position with your shoulders directly above your hands and your hips directly above your knees. In this position it is easier to align your spine optimally. (ii) Keep your spine still, and try to isolate the movement to your abdomen. If you find it hard to stop your spine moving, place a book on your spine to make you more aware of it (tactile feedback).

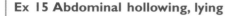

Ex 15 Abdominal hollowing, lying

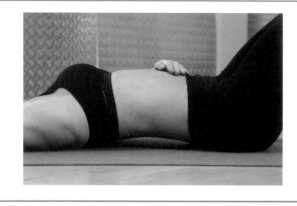
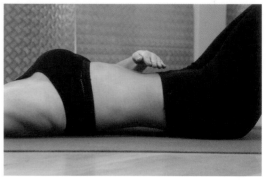

Starting position

Lie on the floor on a mat or towel with your arms either by your sides or folded forwards. Keep your feet comfortably apart. If you are lying on your front, place a folded towel beneath your forehead to avoid squashing your nose.

Action

Perform the abdominal hollowing action by pulling your tummy button inwards and drawing your abdominal wall (tummy surface) off the floor.

Points to note

If you are a little overweight and have a little bit of a 'pot belly', you may not be able to do this exercise! Make sure that you draw your tummy in with abdominal muscle action alone; do not take a deep breath or lift your chest.

Training tip

Train with a partner and lie on a hand towel, folded lengthways, placed under your tummy. As you pull the muscles in tight in the hollowing action, your partner should be able to pull the towel sideways.

Ex 16 Abdominal hollowing, sitting

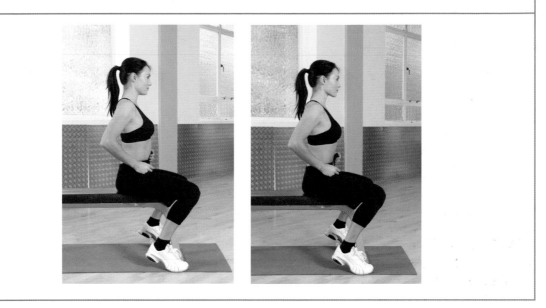

Starting position

Sit on a stool with your knees apart. Sit tall with your back slightly hollow. Place one hand on your tummy and the other in the small of your back.

Action

Perform the abdominal hollowing action by pulling your tummy in and up away from your front hand, focusing your attention on your tummy button.

Points to note

When sitting, try to sit tall, rather than slouching or holding the trunk too rigid.

Training tip

Use your hands to monitor the neutral position of your spine and also to give you feedback about the abdominal hollowing action.

Ex 17 Abdominal hollowing, standing

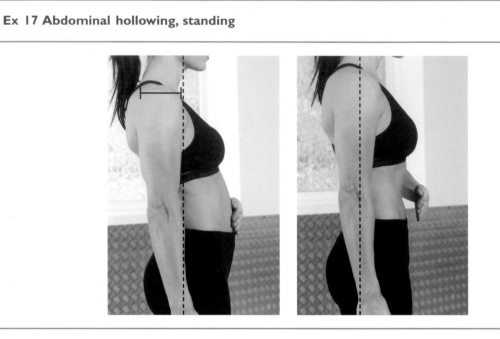

Starting position

Stand upright with your feet shoulder-width apart. Place your lower spine in its neutral position.

Action

Perform the abdominal hollowing action by focusing on your tummy button and pulling it in and up.

Points to note

Breathe normally throughout the movement; do not hold your breath. Make sure that your spine, hips and legs stay still. Isolate the movement to your tummy alone; do not flatten your back or tilt your pelvis.

Training tip

Begin by practising this exercise standing side-on to a mirror. Place a belt loosely around your lower tummy. As you hollow, a gap should form between your tummy and the belt.

Note: The subject begins standing in a sway-back posture. As she performs the exercise her posture is improved and she stands more upright.

Ex 18 Abdominal hollowing, walking

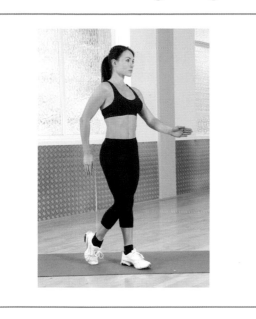

Starting position

Stand upright and perform exercise 17: abdominal hollowing action from standing.

Action

Perform the abdominal hollowing action as you walk for five steps, and then relax your tummy for five steps. Repeat this action for a five-minute walk, breathing normally.

Points to note

As you walk, make sure you do not hold your breath as you are concentrating. Do not breathe too deeply and hyperventilate as this will make you feel lightheaded.

Training tip

If you find you lose control of the coordination of abdominal hollowing and walking, stop, rest and then perform exercise 17: abdominal hollowing, standing once more.

Table 9.1	Common mistakes when performing abdominal hollowing actions		
Mistake	**Noticeable by**	**Reason**	**How to correct**
Ribcage rises	Look at the base of the ribs just above the umbilicus. This should remain on a horizontal line	Subject has taken a deep breath	Place your fingertips on the subject's lower ribs and encourage them to hollow the abdomen while keeping their ribs on your fingers. Instruct the subject to breathe normally
Ribcage depresses	Base of ribcage moves downwards	Subject has activated the rectus abdominis and external oblique muscles	Encourage the subject to put less effort into the hollowing action and to begin the contraction by tightening the pelvis floor
Spine flexes	Back bends and head comes forwards	Subject has activated the rectus abdominis muscle and lost body alignment	Ask the subject to perform the hollowing action while standing with their back against the wall
Breath held	Colour changes in the face. Subject becomes breathless	Subject is not able to disassociate breathing from abdominal hollowing	As the subject hollows the abdomen, ask them to count out loud to ten. Breath-holding then becomes obvious to them

Common mistakes

There are several mistakes which you must take care not to make when performing the abdominal hollowing action. These are outlined above in Table 9.1

Multifidus contraction

The multifidus muscle is important to core stability, especially if you are training your abdominal muscles after back surgery. It is a small muscle at the side of your spine (chapter 2) between the central spinal bones (spinous process) and the large erector muscles. The multifidus lies within the hollow between the spinous process and the erector spinae muscles called the *paraspinal gutter*. It is quite difficult to feel the multifidus, but with practice you should be able to feel a gentle swelling beneath your fingers if you press into the paraspinal gutter. If the muscle is contracting properly, the large erector spinae muscles should remain largely inactive. A good way to check which muscle you are on is to lean forwards slightly (by about 10 degrees) and you should feel the erector spinae muscles standing out like two rigid columns. As you perform multifidus contractions, try to keep the erector spinae relaxed; in other words, you should feel the gentle swelling beneath your fingers without also feeling the rigid column of muscles stand out.

Ex 19 Multifidus setting, sitting

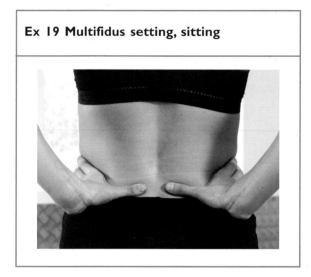

Starting position

Sit at the edge of a stool with your knees and feet shoulder-width apart. Place your thumbs in the small of your back just above waistband level. They should be placed to the side of the bones of your spine (spinous processes), and pressed in to the skin gently.

Action

Gently draw your tummy in (hollowing) and at the same time, press your deep back muscles against your thumbs.

Points to note

The action must be restricted to your deep back muscles. You should not lean or push yourself back, nor hollow or flatten your spine substantially. Only a small local movement of the spinal bones should be felt. Because your knees are apart, you begin with your lower spine slightly hollow. As the multifidus muscle contracts, it will gently deepen the lumbar curve to bring you back towards the neutral back position.

Training tip

Most people find it difficult to feel this muscle contract, so persevere; it is often what you don't feel which is important. As you tighten your back muscles, you should not feel the large columns of muscle at either side of the spine tighten (the erector spinae muscles). Try to focus the muscle action to within 2 cm (1 inch) of the centre of the back. It is helpful to perform a pelvic floor contraction at the same time as tightening the multifidus.

Ex 20 Multifidus setting, standing

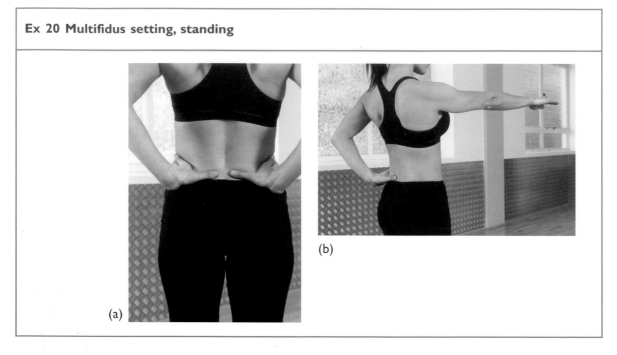

(a)

(b)

Starting position

Stand with your feet apart and place your left thumb into the gap between your spinal bone and the erector muscles of your back on the left hand side (a).

Action

Gently draw your tummy in (hollowing) and see if you can detect your multifidus muscle swelling beneath your fingers. Next, lift your right arm in front of you to the horizontal, keeping it straight (b). Again see if you can feel the multifidus switch on.

Points to note

Try to time the abdominal hollowing and arm lifting together, gently drawing your tummy inwards as your lift your arm.

Training tip

Because multifidus contraction is so subtle, it sometimes helps to close your eyes to really focus your attention on what your fingers are feeling. It can take a couple of training sessions before you feel the muscles switch on so be sure to persevere!

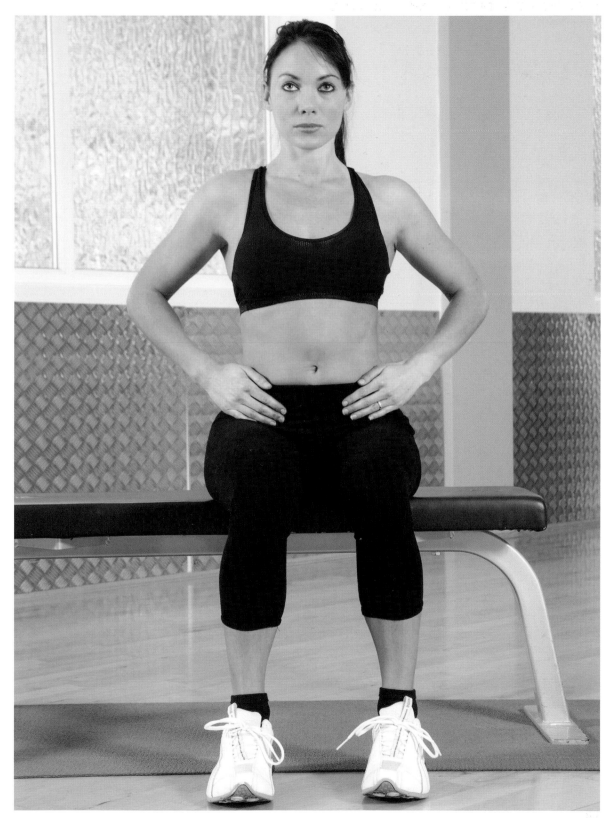

Pelvic floor contractions

The pelvic floor muscles are important to core stability, but they are also important after pregnancy and following surgery of the prostate or bladder. Most women will have been introduced to pelvic floor contraction during pregnancy. Many men, however, are unfamiliar with this type of muscle work, but the pelvic floor is just as important to them. In both sexes, the pelvic floor is important in relation to incontinence and sex life (especially erectile dysfunction in men).

We will look at two pelvic floor exercises. For those who find them difficult, see chapter 14 for details on muscle structure and overcoming contraction difficulties.

Ex 21 Pelvic floor contraction, crook lying

Starting position

Lie on the floor with the knees and feet slightly apart. Relax your buttock muscles (gluteals) and the muscles which pull your legs together (adductors).

Action

Slowly tighten (draw up) the muscles around your back passage (anus). Hold this feeling and try to take it forward to tighten the muscles around the vagina (female) or to lift the penis slightly (male). The feeling should be as though you are trying to stop yourself passing water. Hold for a count of five (breathing normally) and then release.

Points to note

This action is just as important in the male as the female because the pelvic floor muscles work with the deep corset muscles in core stability. In addition, the pelvic floor muscles work to prevent 'dribbling' of urine (incontinence) and to help maintain an erection in the male. Try to perform the action without tensing the gluteal or adductor muscles.

Training tip

Although the action should feel the same as trying to stop the passage of urine, do not perform the action while actually passing urine. This is because this action may interfere with the natural reflexes which control the bladder, making it hard to pass urine in the normal way.

Ex 22 Pelvic floor contraction, sitting

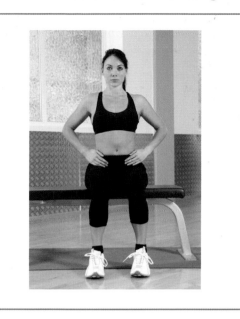

Starting position

Sit on a firm chair or gym bench with your knees and feet slightly apart. Make sure you sit up straight (tall), do not allow yourself to slouch. Relax your buttock muscles (gluteals) and the muscles which pull your legs together (adductors).

Action

Slowly tighten (draw up) the muscles around your back passage (anus). Hold this feeling and try to take it forwards to tighten the muscles around the vagina and pull up inside you (female) or to lift the penis slightly (male). The feeling should be as though you are trying to stop yourself passing water. Hold for a count of 3–5 (breathing normally) and then release.

Points to note

This action is just as important in the male as it is in the female, because the pelvic floor muscles work with the deep corset muscles in core stability. Although the action should feel the same as trying to stop the passage of urine, do not perform the action while actually passing urine – the action may interfere with the natural reflexes which control the bladder, making it hard to pass urine in the normal way.

Training tip

Try to practise the action regularly throughout the day. Tighten the pelvic floor muscles every hour when you are sitting at your desk, or when driving and sitting at the traffic lights for example.

LEVEL ONE

10

The level one exercises build on the stable spine established by the foundation exercises, and introduce forces which challenge the trunk from various angles. In this way, stability becomes more functional. Rather than simply isolating and contracting the stability muscles, we are now using them to protect the spine as we perform increasingly more complex actions. The function of the spine is improved, and with it the cosmetic appearance of the abdominal region.

Ex 23 Heel slide

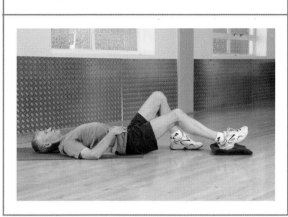

Starting position

Begin lying on the floor on your back. Your feet and knees should be 10–15 cm (4–6 inches) apart. Put your hands on your tummy, with the heel of the hand over your pelvic bones. Place the heel of each foot on a shiny piece of paper on a carpet, or on a soft cloth on a hard wooden floor.

Action

Perform the abdominal hollowing action and hold the abdomen tight. Feel the muscles tense beneath your fingers. Continue to breathe normally throughout the exercise. Slide one leg out straight while holding your tummy tight. As soon as the heel of your hand feels your pelvis begin to tip, slide the leg back in again.

Points to note

The aim of this exercise is to build up the ability of the abdominal muscles to hold the pelvis firm. The action of the leg muscles is therefore secondary to that of the abdominals.

Training tip

The weight of your leg should be taken by the floor throughout the movement. Do not lift your heel up from the ground. The action is to *slide*, not to lift.

Ex 24 Bent knee fallout

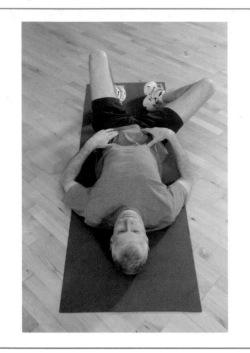

Starting position

Begin lying on the floor on your back with your knees bent and apart by 10–15 cm (4–6 inches) apart. Your feet should be flat on the floor and your arms at about 45 degrees to your body.

Action

Perform the abdominal hollowing action and hold the abdomen tight, breathing normally. Allow your right knee to fall out to the side slowly to 45 degrees and then bring it back to the starting position. Repeat the action with the left knee.

Points to note

The aim of this exercise is to improve the ability of the abdominal muscles to hold the lumbar spine firm. The action of the leg muscles is therefore secondary to that of the abdominals.

Training tip

The weight of your leg should be taken by the floor throughout the movement: do not lift your foot.

Ex 25 Leg shortening, lying

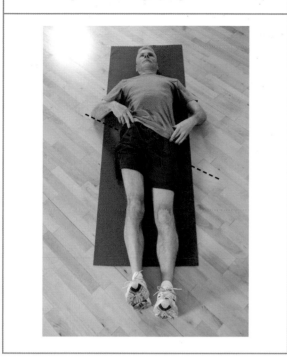

Starting position

Begin lying on the floor on your back with your feet 20 cm (8 inches) apart. Place your arms out sideways in a 'T' shape or use your hands to monitor your pelvis.

Action

Move your pelvis up and down at the side ('hitching the hip') to shorten and then lengthen each leg.

Points to note

The leg must remain perfectly straight to focus the movement on the pelvis and, through this, on to the lower spine.

Training tip

Flex your foot, and lead the movement with your heel.

Ex 26 Side lying, spine lengthening

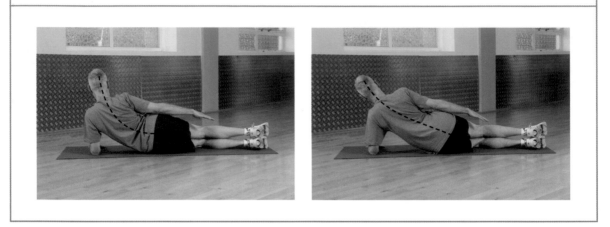

Starting position

Lie on your side with your knees together and slightly bent. Prop yourself up on one elbow so that your back is gently curved.

Action

Tighten (hollow) your tummy and lift the lower side of the trunk upwards so that you straighten your spine. Hold the position for 5 seconds and then lower.

Points to note

Hollowing tightens the muscles at the front and sides of your tummy, while this exercise tightens the side muscles still further. The result is that you feel improved muscle tone around the whole of your waist.

Training tip

Do not lift the underneath hip, simply allow it to rock gently on the floor as you straighten the spine.

Ex 27 Plank

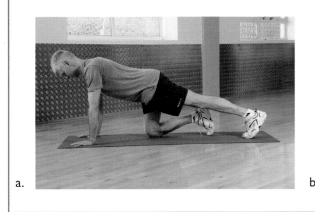

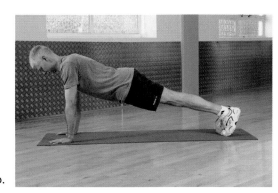

a.

b.

Starting position

Begin kneeling on all fours (four point kneeling).

Action

Tighten (hollow) your tummy and lock your arms fully. Straighten first one (a) and then the other leg, taking your weight on the balls of your feet (b). Hold the position for 5–10 seconds and then lower.

Points to note

You should aim to form a straight line through your feet, knees, hips, and shoulders. If you are unable to maintain this line, and your hips drop, stop the exercise and re-start.

Training tip

If you find the alignment of this exercise difficult, ask a training partner to lift your pelvis and place you into a straight line. Begin holding for 2–3 seconds and build up to the full 10 seconds.

Ex 28 Abdominal hollowing and leg straightening

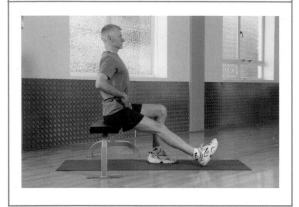

Starting position

Sit on a chair or stool with your feet off the ground. Tighten (hollow) your abdomen and sit up straight, lengthening your spine.

Action

Keep your tummy muscles tight (hollow) and gradually straighten one leg, maintaining your normal back alignment.

Points to note

When you straighten one leg, tension in the hamstring muscles at the back of the leg will pull on your sitting bone (*ishial tuberosity*) and try to tilt your pelvis backwards, rounding your lower back. Ensure you maintain your alignment and prevent this.

Training tip

If your training partner places their hand about 1–2 cm (½ inch) behind the small of your back, they will be able to monitor the lumbar hollow (lordosis) and tell you if your alignment is being maintained.

Ex 29 Leg lowering, supine

Starting position

Lie on the floor with your feet comfortably apart. Place your fingertips on either side of your tummy below the level of your tummy button.

Action

Tighten (hollow) your abdomen and hold it tight throughout the exercise. Raise one leg (keeping it straight) to a count of one, to 30–45 degrees above the horizontal. Pause in this position and then lower the raised leg back to the floor to a count of five. Rest in the lying position for 2 seconds and then repeat with the other leg.

Points to note

On no account should both legs move together. Do not lift the second leg until the first is back on the floor and you have rested for 2 seconds. If you find the exercise too hard, bend both knees and lift the leg with the knee bent. This will shorten the leg lever and make the exercise easier.

Training tip

Monitor the position of your tummy with your fingertips. If you feel your tummy bulging ('ballooning') rather than staying flat, stop the exercise.

Ex 30 Trunk curl shoulder lift

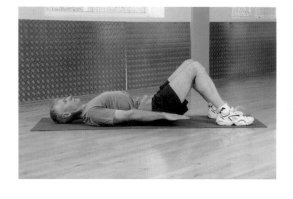 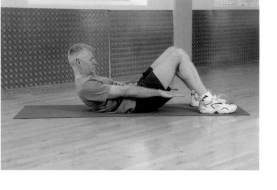

Starting position

Begin lying on your back with your knees bent. Your feet should be shoulder-width apart.

Action

Perform the abdominal hollowing action, pulling your tummy button in. Reach forwards with your fingers towards your heels so that your trunk bends and your shoulders lift slightly away from the floor. Your lower back should press lightly towards the mat.

Points to note

The action of this exercise is to bend the trunk, not to lift it from the mat. The bottom part of the shoulder blades should stay in contact with the ground throughout the movement. As you perform the abdominal hollowing action, breathe out. Breathe in as you release the movement.

Training tip

Reaching forwards (along the ground) towards the heels, rather than upwards for the knees, encourages the correct trunk bending action.

Ex 31 V sit stage 1

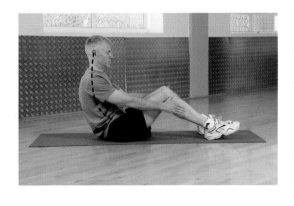 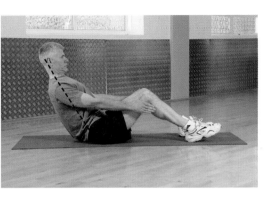

Starting position

Sit on a gym mat with your knees hip-width apart and bent, feet flat (the crook or hook sitting position). Place your hands to the outsides of your knees palms facing inwards.

Action

Tighten your tummy muscles and lean back slightly to straighten your back, bracing your shoulders. Straighten your arms and hold this 'V' shaped body position, breathing normally.

Points to note

You will finish the movement sitting on three points forming a tripod – both sitting bones (ischial tuberosities) and your tailbone (coccyx). If you find this painful, you may not have enough padding from the mat so sit on a folded towel placed on top of your mat.

Training tip

Your spine should be correctly aligned, with a gentle lumbar (low back) curve, breastbone lifted, shoulder blades drawn back and down slightly and thoracic (upper) back almost straight. Avoid an excessive spinal curve into extension (hyperextension) or flexion (spine rounding).

Ex 32 Lying posterior pelvic tilt

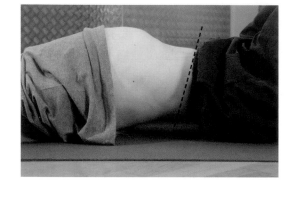 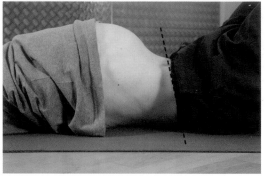

Starting position

Begin lying on your back with your knees bent, feet shoulder-width apart.

Action

Abdominal hollow and then tilt your pelvis backwards flattening your back on to the floor. Hold the position for 3 seconds and release.

Points to note

Keep your buttocks on the mat as you perform this action.

Training tip

As you perform the pelvic tilt, think about pointing your pubic bone towards your head and, as you release the action, point it away. It sometimes helps to visualise a saucer of water resting on your tummy. As you tilt your pelvis posteriorly, imagine that you are tipping the water onto your lower ribs.

Ex 33 Abdominal hollowing with gluteal brace

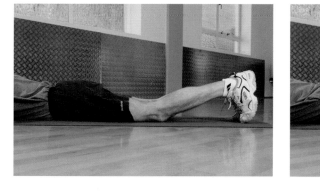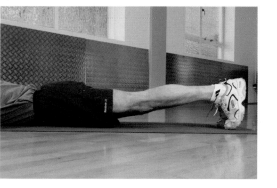

Starting position

Begin lying on your front on the floor. Tuck your feet under so your toes are bent (flexed). Place a folded towel beneath your forehead for comfort.

Action

Perform the abdominal hollowing action by pulling your tummy in tight, focusing your attention on your tummy button. At the same time, tighten your buttocks and brace your legs out straight.

Points to note

You must maintain the neutral position of your spine throughout the action. Make sure you don't tilt your pelvis forwards or backwards.

Training tip

Tighten your tummy first, and then grip your buttocks together. Once you have mastered the individual actions, try performing both at the same time.

Ex 34 Pelvic shift and knee unload

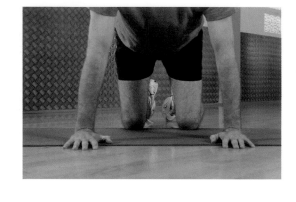
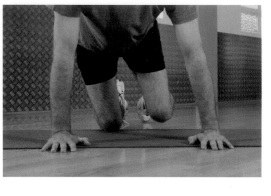

Starting position

Begin kneeling on your hands and knees (four-point kneeling). Your knees should be hip-width apart, your hands shoulder-width apart.

Action

Perform the abdominal hollowing action and shift your pelvis to the right, taking most of your weight through your right knee. Slightly (1cm) lift your left knee clear of the mat. Maintain the position for 2–5 seconds and then lower the left knee onto the mat. Repeat the action to the right.

Points to note

Because you lift your left knee barely clear of the mat, your hips should stay more or less in line. If you lift your knees too high, you will twist your spine.

Training tip

Placing a book on your lower back can help you feel the subtle movement of the pelvis.

Ex 35 Kneeling single leg lift

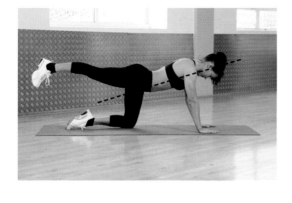 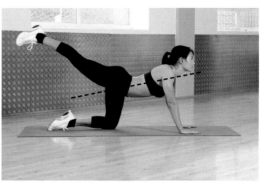

Starting position

Begin kneeling on your hands and knees (four-point kneeling). Your knees should be hip-width apart, your hands shoulder-width apart.

Action

Shift your pelvis to the left taking most of your weight on your left knee. Lift your right knee just clear of the mat. Straighten your right leg to the horizontal position. Hold the straight position for 2 seconds and then lower the leg. Repeat on your left leg.

Points to note

As you straighten the leg, make sure you don't twist your spine.

Training tip

The action is to lengthen the leg as well as lift it. If you find you are losing good alignment, have a training partner gently pull on your foot to encourage the leg lengthening action.

Note: The subject has lifted her leg too high, causing her spine to arch. Lift the leg to the horizontal only.

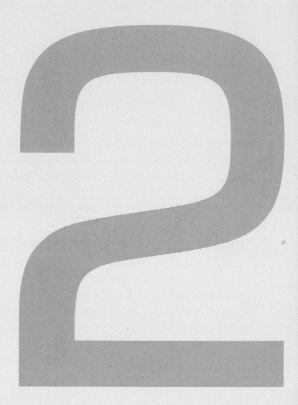

LEVEL TWO

11

The level two exercises continue the job of the level one programme and build an increasingly greater variety of movements. Overall trunk fitness is improved by further enhancing stability and building upon strength, endurance and skill.

Ex 36 Trunk curl sequence

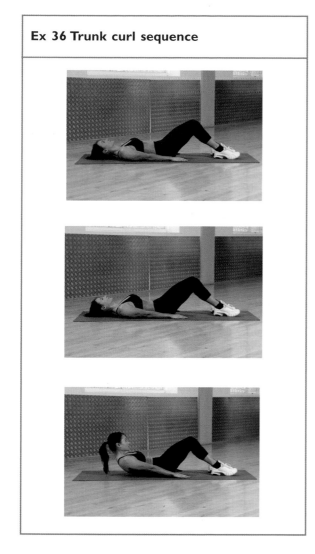

Starting position

Begin lying on your back with your knees bent. Your feet should be shoulder-width apart.

Action

Perform the pelvic tilt and flatten your back onto the floor. Next, perform the abdominal hollowing action, pulling your tummy button in. Finally, reach forwards with your fingers towards your heels so that your trunk bends and your shoulders lift from the floor.

Points to note

The action of this exercise is to bend the trunk, not to sit up. The bottom part of the shoulder blades should stay in contact with the ground throughout the movement. As you perform the abdominal hollowing action, breathe out. Breathe in as you release the movement.

Training tip

Reaching forwards (along the ground) towards the heels, rather than upwards for the knees, encourages the correct trunk bending action.

Ex 37 X tone

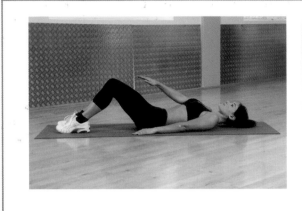
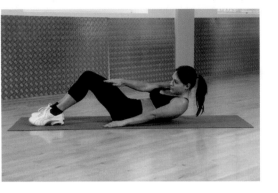

Starting position

Begin lying on the floor on your back with your knees bent, feet flat. Your knees and feet should be about 20–30 cm (8–12 inches) apart.

Action

Abdominal hollow to tighten your abdominal muscles, and then reach past the outside of your left knee with your right hand. At the same time, pull the left side of your pelvis towards you. Pause and then reverse the action, reaching to the right.

Points to note

The aim of this exercise is to tone the oblique abdominals. To achieve this, the lower part of the trunk must take part in the action, so the hip pull is essential to the exercise.

Training tip

To emphasise the hip pull action, initially ask someone to press onto your hip as you pull. This will make isolating the action easier. Remember to lift only one hip at a time!

Ex 38 Single bent leg lowering from crunch position

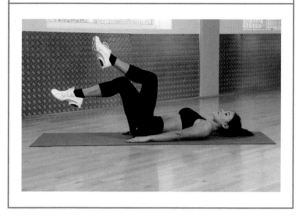

Starting position

Lie on the floor and draw your knees up to rest above your hips – feet off the floor – moving one knee at a time. You can place your fingertips on either side of your lower abdomen below your tummy button to feel the muscle contraction.

Action

Tighten your tummy muscles to hollow your abdomen, and maintain this muscle contraction throughout the exercise. Slowly lower one leg, keeping it bent, until your foot touches the floor. Raise the leg and, when it is in the starting position again, begin to lower the other leg.

Points to note

The foot should be lowered directly downwards, keeping it close to the buttocks. Do not allow the leg to straighten as this makes the exercise considerably more intense.

Training tip

Monitor the position of your tummy and pelvis with your fingertips. If you feel your tummy bulging ('ballooning') rather than staying flat, or if you feel your pelvis move, stop the exercise.

Ex 39 V sit stage 2

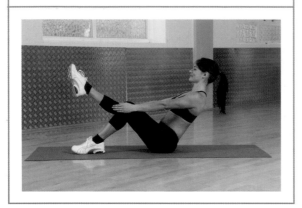

Starting position

Sit on the floor with your knees hip-width apart and bent, and feet flat (the crook or hook sitting position). Straighten your back, bracing your shoulders back slightly into the V sit position (exercise 31, page 111). Hold your arms to the sides of your knees, palms facing inwards.

Action

Tighten your tummy muscles to hollow your abdomen, and maintain this muscle contraction throughout the exercise. Straighten your right leg keeping your left foot firmly on the floor. Hold the straight leg position for 5 seconds and then lower. Repeat the action with the left leg.

Points to note

As you straighten your leg, maintain the hip angle so that the leg is held at 45 degrees to the mat. Lowering the leg towards the mat increases the leverage effect on the leg and makes the action considerably harder.

Training tip

There is often a tendency to bend (flex) the spine with this action. Try to maintain good spinal alignment throughout the exercise.

Ex 40 Pelvic raise (1)

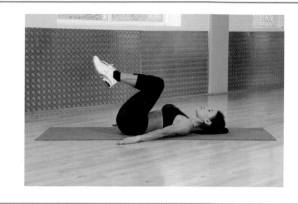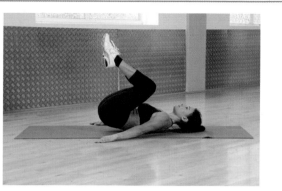

Starting position

Begin lying on the floor on your back. Your arms should rest on the floor by your sides (palms down) making an angle of 45 degrees to your body. Bend your knees and draw them up onto your chest.

Action

Bend your spine to lift your tailbone 3 cm (1 inch) off the ground, at the same time pulling your knees upwards towards your shoulders.

Points to note

Do not lunge into the movement using the momentum of your legs. The action should be a gentle raising of the lower spine, with the power of the trunk muscles lifting the inactive legs.

Training tip

Press down hard with your straight arms onto the floor as you flex your lower spine. If you find you are unable to lift your body, reach your arms overhead to hold on to a piece of gym machinery. Be cautious, however, because by fixing the arms in this way you are able to lift your body further – keep your mid-back on the floor.

Ex 41 Bench crunch

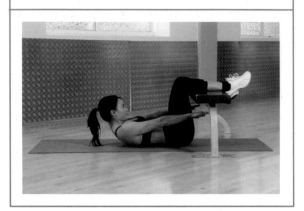

Starting position

Begin lying on the floor on your back. Place your calves on a low chair or stool so that your knees and hips are bent to 90 degrees. Your feet and knees should be 20–30 cm (8–12 inches) apart.

Action

Slowly sit forwards, as though trying to touch your chest flat onto your thighs.

Points to note

This is an advanced exercise and, as such, you may not be able to lift very far forwards to begin with. Do not speed the movement up in an attempt to sit up further. This will simply increase the momentum of your trunk, but will not work the abdominal muscles substantially harder.

Training tip

Try to bend your trunk as you begin to sit forwards, to shorten the abdominal muscles.

Ex 42 Oblique bench crunch

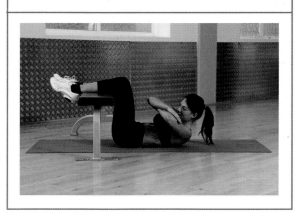

Do not attempt this exercise until you can comfortably perform ten repetitions of exercise 41: bench crunch (page 122).

Starting position

Begin lying on the floor on your back. Place your calves on a low chair or stool so that your knees and hips are bent to 90 degrees. Your feet and knees should be 20–30 cm (8–12 inches) apart. Fold your arms lightly, keeping your elbows bent to 90 degrees.

Action

Sit up, and at the same time reach your right elbow past your left knee. Lower back to the floor and repeat the action, reaching with your left elbow past your right knee.

Points to note

As with the bench crunch, make sure that the exercise is performed slowly, under control. A rapid action will enable you to sit up further, but only through momentum.

Training tip

Exhale as you sit up, but rest after each pair of oblique crunches, and breathe normally so you do not get dizzy.

Ex 43 Knee rolling

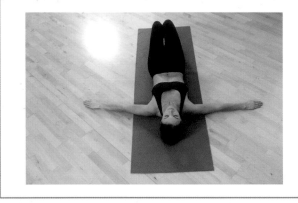
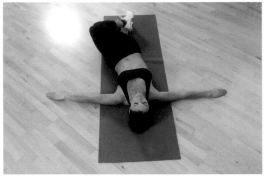

Starting position

Lie on your back with your knees bent, feet flat on the floor (crook lying position). Place your arms out sideways in a 'T' shape to aid stability.

Action

Allow your knees to lower slowly to one side, forming an angle of about 30 degrees to the vertical. Pull the knees back to the mid-position and then repeat the action.

Points to note

Breathe normally throughout the exercise; do not hold your breath. Make sure you keep both feet on the ground as you lower the knees.

Training tip

If you cannot lower your knees to the ground, place a cushion on the floor at either side of your hips. Lower your knees onto the cushion to begin with, rather than right down onto the floor.

Ex 44 Bridging

Starting position

Begin lying on your back with your knees bent and feet flat on the floor (crook lying position). Your feet should be shoulder-width apart. Find the neutral position of your back and maintain this throughout the exercise.

Action

Perform the abdominal hollowing action and then tighten your buttock muscles and lift your hips 10 cm (4 inches) from the floor.

Points to note

The lower spine must stay in its neutral position, so make sure that you don't lift too high or your spine will arch. Your shoulder, hip and upper leg should be in line.

Training tip

Allow the squeeze of the buttock muscles to lead the movement and lift you, rather than leading with your stomach.

Ex 45 Bridging on a gym ball

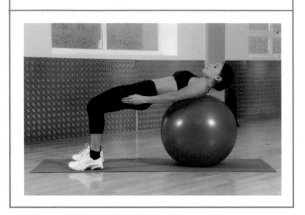

Starting position

Lie with your shoulders on a gym ball and your feet shoulder-width apart.

Action

Tighten (hollow) your tummy and raise your hips from the floor to the horizontal position. Hold this position for 3–5 seconds and then slowly lower.

Points to note

You must make sure that you keep your tummy tight throughout the action and avoid allowing your back to hollow excessively.

Training tip

If you find it difficult to lift into the position, begin with your hips on a block or low stool and raise from here. The gym ball is an unstable surface and this makes your trunk muscles work harder to maintain your own core stability. However, until you get used to the exercise you can stop the ball from rolling by placing it on a ball ring, available from gym ball suppliers.

Note: The gym ball is slightly too large for the subject. Try to use a ball which is the same height as your knee.

Ex 46 Side-lying body lift

Starting position

Lie on your side on a gym mat. Place your feet together and keep your legs straight. Prop yourself up on your underneath forearm, and tighten (hollow) your abdomen.

Action

Raise your body so that your spine is straight and you are just balanced on your feet and underneath forearm.

Points to note

The underneath side trunk muscles (obliques) are working in this exercise together with your deep corset muscles.

Training tip

Make sure you broaden your shoulders as you lift so that you don't feel that they are 'bunched up'. If you perform this exercise in bare feet, place your top foot in front of your bottom foot.

Ex 47 Ab frame crunch

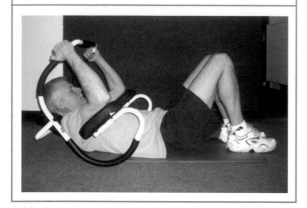

Starting position

Lie on a mat with your knees bent and slightly apart. Place your hands on the handles of the ab frame and your head on the headrest. Tighten (hollow) your abdomen.

Action

Curl the trunk while resting your head gently on the machine head-rest. Hold for 1–2 seconds in the upper position breathing normally, and then slowly lower.

Points to note

The aim of the ab frame is to assist the movement and maintain good alignment. Make sure that you keep your head on the headrest and use only enough hand pressure on the frame to enable you to perform the action smoothly. If you find yourself pushing back hard onto the headrest, allow your neck and upper spine to bend a little and look through your knees.

Training tip

As you get tired, you will need to use more hand pressure on the frame. When this happens, make sure that you keep the movement slow and controlled, avoiding any jerking actions.

Ex 48 Kneeling leg and arm raise

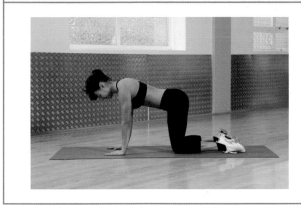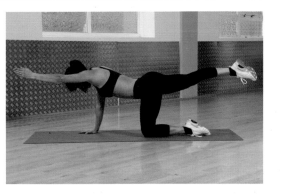

Starting position

Begin kneeling on a mat with your shoulder directly above your hand and your hip directly above your knee. Tighten (hollow) your abdomen.

Action

Raise your right leg to the horizontal. Hold this position and then raise your left arm towards the horizontal. Hold the arm/leg position for 3–5 seconds and then lower. Repeat the action using your left leg and right arm.

Points to note

Make sure you maintain the neutral position of your spine and a gentle tightness in your abdominal muscles throughout the action. Do not allow your spine to sag or your tummy to 'balloon'. This exercise is also called the 'birdog'.

Training tip

If your shoulder is quite tight, you may not be able to lift your arm to the horizontal initially. With practice, your arm will lift higher as you gain shoulder flexibility.

LEVEL THREE

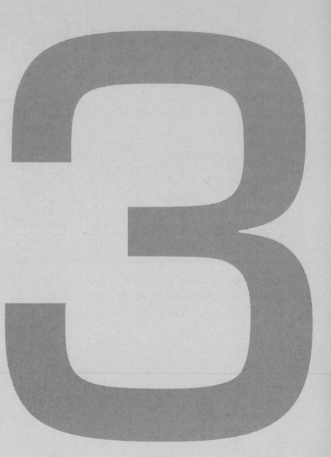

Up to this point we have used 48 abdominal training exercises. For the most part these are all that is required for everyday trunk fitness. For those who need greater levels of function we now look at level three exercises, which are harder still. Maintain good technique, however, paying particular attention to alignment and maintaining back stability.

Ex 49 Single straight leg lowering from crunch position

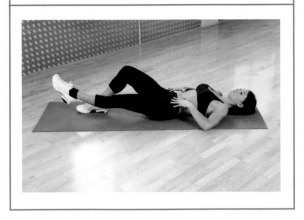

Do not attempt this exercise until you can perform ten repetitions of exercise 38: single bent leg lowering from crunch position (page 119), maintaining a neutral position of the lumbar spine throughout the exercise.

Starting position

Lie on the floor with your knees bent and feet flat. Draw your right knee up above your hip, and straighten your left leg resting it on the floor.

Action

Tighten your tummy muscles to hollow your abdomen, and maintain this muscle contraction throughout the exercise. Keep your right (bent) leg still, and slowly lift and lower your left (straight) leg, maintaining the neutral position of your lumbar spine.

Points to note

Lifting the leg higher reduces the leverage effect of the straight leg and so makes the exercise easier from the point of the abdominal muscles.

Training tip

Monitor the position of your tummy and pelvis with your fingertips. If you feel your tummy bulging ('ballooning') rather than staying flat, or if you feel your pelvis move, stop the exercise.

Ex 50 V sit stage 3

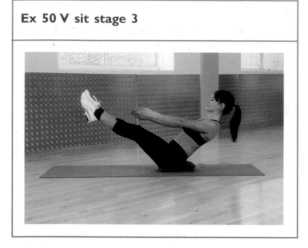

Do not attempt this exercise until you can comfortably perform five repetitions with each leg of exercise 39: V sit stage 2 (page 120).

Starting position

Sit on the floor with your knees hip-width apart and bent, and feet flat (the crook or hook sitting position). Place your straight arms to the sides of your knees, palms facing inwards. Straighten your back, bracing your shoulders back slightly into the V sit position (exercise 31, page 111).

Action

Tighten your tummy muscles to hollow your abdomen slightly, and maintain this muscle contraction throughout the exercise. Straighten your right leg, keeping your left foot firmly on the floor. Hold the right leg straight and then straighten the left leg, pulling the legs together. Hold for 5 seconds and then lower.

Points to note

As you straighten your legs, maintain the hip angle so that the leg is held at 45 degrees to the mat. Lowering the legs towards the mat increases the leverage effect on the leg and makes the action considerably harder, placing excessive stress on the lumbar spine.

Training tip

There is often a tendency to bend (flex) the spine with this action. Try to maintain good spinal alignment throughout the exercise. A useful cue is to imagine a cord attached to your breastbone (*sternum*) pulling your chest forwards. In the end position, your straight legs and trunk should form a full 'V' shape. In yoga this exercise is called the boat pose (*navasana*).

Ex 51 Russian twist

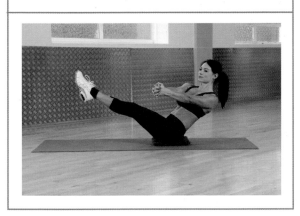

Starting position

Lie on the floor and bend your knees. Lift your legs, keeping them bent, and keep your feet off the floor throughout the exercise. Sit up, with your hands together and your trunk off the ground forming a 'V' shape (*see* exercise 31, page 111).

Action

Reach your arms out straight, and twist your trunk to the left, then right, leading with your hands.

Points to note

You should remain balanced on your sitting bones (ishial tuberosities) and tailbone (*coccyx*) throughout the exercise.

Training tip

If you find the action too intense, allow your heels to just touch the floor as you twist your trunk.

Ex 52 Trunk twist holding disc

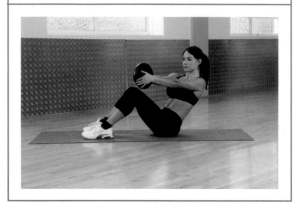

Starting position

Lie on the floor and bend your knees, keeping your feet flat and shoulder-width apart. Sit up, holding a 5 kg weight disc at its edge.

Action

Reach your arms out straight, and twist your trunk to the left, and then right, leading with your hands.

Points to note

You should remain balanced on your sitting bones (ishial tuberosities) throughout the exercise, and your feet should stay on the mat.

Training tip

Choose a weight which suits your body size and strength. Make sure you perform the exercise correctly rather than using a weight which is too heavy – there is an old weight training adage 'never sacrifice technique for weight!'

Ex 53 Pelvic raise (2)

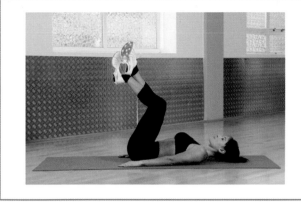 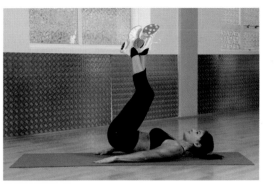

You must be able to perform 5–10 repetitions of exercise 40: pelvic raise 1, page 121, before attempting this exercise.

Starting position

Begin lying on the floor on your back. Your arms should rest on the floor by your sides (palms down), making an angle of 45 degrees to your body. Bend your knees and hips to 90 degrees (crunch position).

Action

Bend your spine to lift your tailbone 3 cm (1 inch) off the ground, while holding your hips completely still.

Points to note

This exercise works the lower abdominals hard. However, work is taken off these muscles if rapid hip flexion is used to lever the spine off the floor. The hips should stay inactive throughout the movement, with the power of the exercise coming from the lower abdominals only. Keep the knees off the chest.

Training tip

Press down hard with your straight arms onto the floor as you flex your lower spine. Begin by lifting the tailbone and then the last spinal bone followed by the next to last. If you find you are unable to lift your body, reach your arms overhead to hold onto a piece of gym machinery. Be cautious, however, because by fixing the arms in this way you are able to lift your body further – keep your mid-back on the floor.

Ex 54 Side bend in side lying

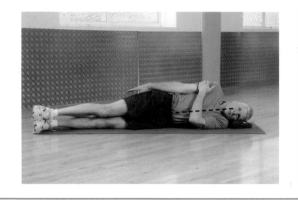
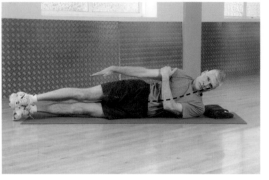

Starting position

Begin lying on your side on a mat. Bend your lower arm and leg slightly to improve your stability. Rest your head lightly on a towel for support.

Action

Perform a side-bending action so that your lower shoulder lifts from the floor by 2 cm (¾ inch). At the same time, 'hitch' your upper leg to shorten it by 2 cm (¾ inch).

Points to note

The side-bend movement is very small so neither the trunk nor the leg should lift far.

Training tip

Imagine you are 'gathering' the skin at the side of the trunk as your trunk pulls in one direction and your leg in the other.

Ex 55 Rope climb

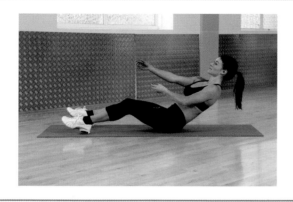 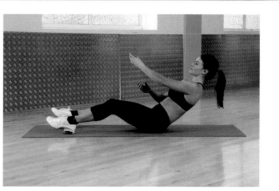

Do not attempt this exercise until you can perform ten repetitions of exercise 36: trunk curl (page 117) and exercise 41: bench crunch (page 122) comfortably.

Starting position

Begin lying on the floor with your knees bent, arms by your sides. Your feet and knees should be 20–30 cm (8–12 inches) apart.

Action

Imagine a line joining your knees, and focus on a point just above the centre of this line. Reach up with your right hand for this point by curling and twisting your trunk. Pause and then allow yourself to sit back down partially. Immediately reach up with the other hand to the same point and then repeat the action.

Points to note

The lower spine should stay on the ground; only the chest and shoulders lift up. Keep the trunk curled throughout the movement so that you maintain tension in the abdominal muscles. Make sure your chin is tucked in; do not allow your chin to poke forwards and lead the movement. Breathe normally; do not hold your breath.

Training tip

As you reach towards the high point in this movement, grip as though you are pulling on a rope. As you lower down, keep reaching forwards with your arm to maintain the curled position of the trunk.

Ex 56 Barbell rollout

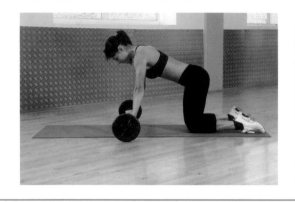 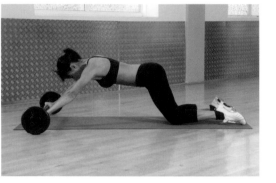

Do not attempt this exercise until you can perform 10 repetitions of exercise 27: the plank (page 107), comfortably.

Starting position

Begin kneeling, hands holding a barbell placed in front of you. Your feet and knees should be 20–30 cm (8–12 inches) apart.

Action

Slowly roll the barbell forwards, lowering your body from a kneeling position to a press-up position (prone fall). Hold this position for 1–2 seconds and then roll the barbell back and move into the kneeling position again.

Points to note

The exercise gets harder the further out you roll the barbell, and the longer your hold the end point of the plank position.

Training tip

Begin just rolling the bar forwards so that your arms are at 45 degrees to the vertical. Once you are used to this, reach further forwards.

Ex 57 Negative crunch

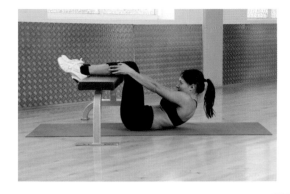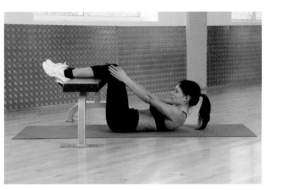

Do not attempt this exercise until you can perform ten repetitions of exercise 41: bench crunch (page 122), comfortably.

Starting position

Begin lying on a mat on your back. Place your calves on a low chair or stool so that your knees and hips are bent to 90 degrees. Your feet and knees should be 20–30 cm (8–12 inches) apart. Fix your feet by hooking them under an object or ask a training partner to hold them firmly.

Action

Reach forwards and grip your knees. Pull yourself up using just arm strength until your chest touches your thighs. Flex your trunk so that your head touches your knees, and maintain this flexed position throughout the exercise. Slowly lower your upper body back down onto the floor inch by inch, taking a total of 30 seconds to complete the entire movement (eccentric muscle action).

Points to note

Make sure you breathe normally throughout the movement; do not hold your breath.

Training tip

Ensure that your tail touches the floor first, followed by the small of your back, the mid-back, shoulder blades and finally the shoulders.

Ex 58 Straight leg roll

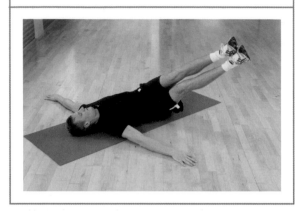

Do not attempt this exercise until you can perform ten repetitions of exercise 43: knee rolling (page 124) comfortably.

Starting position

Lie on the floor with your knees bent. Stretch your arms out to the side in a 'T' shape to aid stability. Draw your knees up onto your chest then straighten your legs so that your hips, knees and feet are in line, and you form a 90 degree angle at your waist.

Action

Gradually lower your legs, keeping them straight, sideways onto the floor. Keep the arms and shoulders pressed tightly against the floor for stability.

Points to note

The hips remain on the floor as the trunk twists. Make sure the action stays controlled. Do not allow the legs to drop rapidly to the floor.

Training tip

When you begin the exercise, place two cushions on the floor at either side of your hips. Start the exercise by lowering your legs onto the cushions rather than the floor.

Ex 59 Double leg hold using gym ball

Starting position

Begin in the press-up position with your thighs on a gym ball. Your hands should be slightly wider than shoulder-width apart. Tighten (hollow) your tummy muscles and hold them tight throughout the exercise.

Action

Keep your legs straight and horizontal, and walk your hands backwards towards the ball so the ball moves up your body to your waist. Hold this position for 3–5 seconds and then walk your hands back to the starting position.

Points to note

The aim of this exercise is to maintain alignment by tensing the abdomen, buttock, and back muscles. A balanced contraction between these muscle groups is required without one muscle group dominating. It is essential, therefore, that the body is in line; the legs should not be extended above the horizontal and the back should not hollow excessively.

Training tip

To begin with, walk the arms towards the ball until the ball rests at knee level. Once this is comfortable, walk the arms further until the ball rests at the hips. Finally, walk the arms so that the ball rests at the waist. In this way the exercise intensity is increased gradually (progressively).

Ex 60 Gym ball leg roll

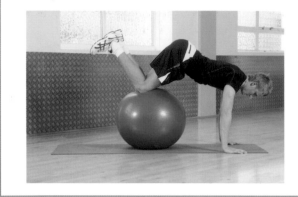 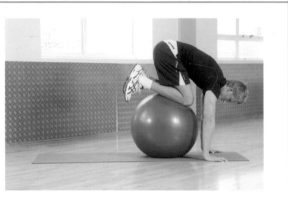

Starting position

Begin in the press-up position with your knees on a gym ball. Your hands should be slightly wider than shoulder-width apart and your body kept straight; you should not allow your hips to sag.

Action

Draw your feet towards you, rolling your legs over the ball until you touch the ball with your feet. Pause in this position and then roll your feet out again.

Points to note

When you begin the exercise make sure that your body is straight. The knees, hips and shoulders should form a line.

Training tip

As you draw your feet towards your hands, your hips will lift above the level of your shoulders.

Ex 61 Ab frame reverse crunch

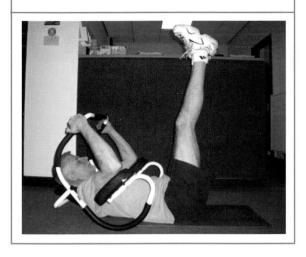

Do not use this exercise until you can perform ten repetitions of exercise 47: ab frame crunch (page 128) comfortably.

Starting position

Lie on the floor with your knees bent. Place your head on the headrest of the ab frame and hold onto the handle. Tighten (hollow) your tummy and then lift first one leg to the vertical position, and then the other. Make sure you keep your knee bent as you lift the leg and straighten it only when the knee is above the hip.

Action

Keep the upper body still and slowly lift your legs as though you were trying to touch the ceiling with your toes. Hold the upper position for 1–2 seconds then slowly lower.

Points to note

The action is to tilt the pelvis backwards by flattening the back against the floor and then to lift the tailbone.

Training tip

There is very little movement involved with this exercise. Aim to lift the waistband of your shorts about 2 cm (1 inch) from the floor.

Ex 62 Ab frame oblique crunch

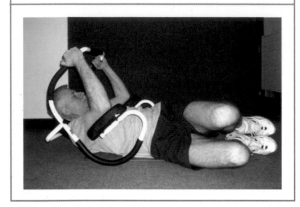

Starting position

Begin lying on a mat with your knees bent and slightly apart. Place your hands on the handles of the ab frame and your head on the headrest. Tighten (hollow) your abdomen, and lower your knees to the right to rest on the mat.

Action

Lower you knees to the right. Curl the trunk while resting your head gently on the machine headrest. Hold for 1–2 seconds in the upper position breathing normally, and then slowly lower. Perform five repetitions with your knees resting on the right-hand side and then repeat the action for five reps with your knees resting on the left.

Points to note

The aim of the ab frame is to assist the movement and maintain good alignment. Make sure that you keep your head on the headrest and use only enough hand pressure on the frame to enable you to perform the action smoothly. If you find yourself pushing back hard onto the headrest, allow your neck and upper spine to bend a little and look through your knees.

Training tip

As you get tired, you will need to use more hand pressure on the frame. When this happens, make sure that you keep the movement slow and controlled, avoiding any jerking actions.

Ex 63 Controlled straight leg sit-up

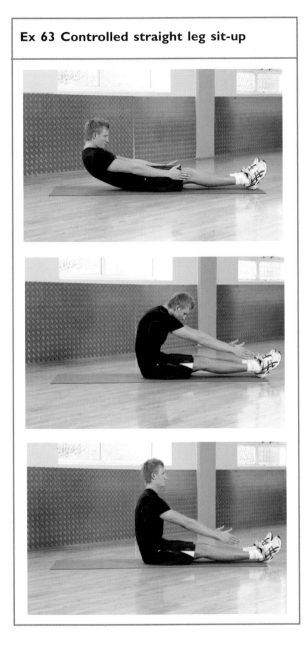

Starting position

Begin lying on your back with your legs straight, hands by your sides.

Action

Perform the abdominal hollowing action and then reach forwards with your fingers towards the outsides of your knees so that your trunk bends and your shoulders lift from the floor. Continue the movement until you sit up completely. Pause in the sitting position and then slowly lower back down to lying by bending your trunk and lowering firstly the low back, followed by the mid-back and then the upper back.

Points to note

The action of this exercise is to bend the trunk to reduce the leverage effect of the spine and effectively make it lighter. If you can achieve this, the legs will not lift. If your legs do begin to lift, stop immediately, as the exercise is not suitable for you.

Training tip

Reaching forwards (along the ground) towards the outside of the knees, rather than upwards above the knees, encourages the correct trunk bending action.

ABDOMINAL TRAINING IN SPORT AND EXERCISE CLASSES

13

The principles which make up this abdominal training programme may be used in sport in two ways. Firstly, the exercises described in the earlier chapters may be incorporated into a general training programme. This will have the effect of making the trunk section of any training programme far safer and more effective. In addition, because the arms and legs depend on the stability of the trunk as the core against which they push and pull, the function of the limbs may well improve. Finally, the programme can contribute by using the underlying principle of enhanced trunk stability to provide the foundation for movements in all sports actions. The following exercises demonstrate a few examples of how commonly used exercises can be modified using core stability principles to improve both safety and effectiveness.

> ## Keypoint
>
> Using core stability principles can make your sport both safer and more effective.

Weight training

We have seen that the neutral position of the spine should be maintained as often as possible to reduce stress acting on the lumbar region. One way to achieve this, and stabilise the spine is to practise the abdominal hollowing action. By pulling abdominal muscles in tightly, the trunk becomes more stable and body alignment

is improved. In fig. 13.1a, the athlete is performing a shoulder press action. The pelvis has tipped forwards and the lumbar curve has become excessive. By tightening the abdominal muscles (*see* fig. 13.1b), the pelvis will remain level and the lumbar spine is correctly aligned. In addition, the athlete in fig. 13.1b has widened the base of support and is therefore more stable. The combination of stable spine and stable base makes the exercise far safer.

The same applies to fig. 13.2. Initially, the athlete performing the arm curl has allowed the pelvis to tip forwards and is dangerously overextending (hyperextending) the spine to swing the weight upwards. In fig. 13.2b, by modifying the exercise using the programme's principles, the exercise is far safer. Firstly, posture modification and abdominal hollowing has been used to correct the pelvic tilt and give the athlete a stable trunk to work from. Secondly, the base of support has been widened by placing the feet one in front of the other, and the knees are bent so that the legs, rather than the spine, give the spring to the action.

> ## Keypoint
>
> When using weights, focus on good body alignment throughout each movement.

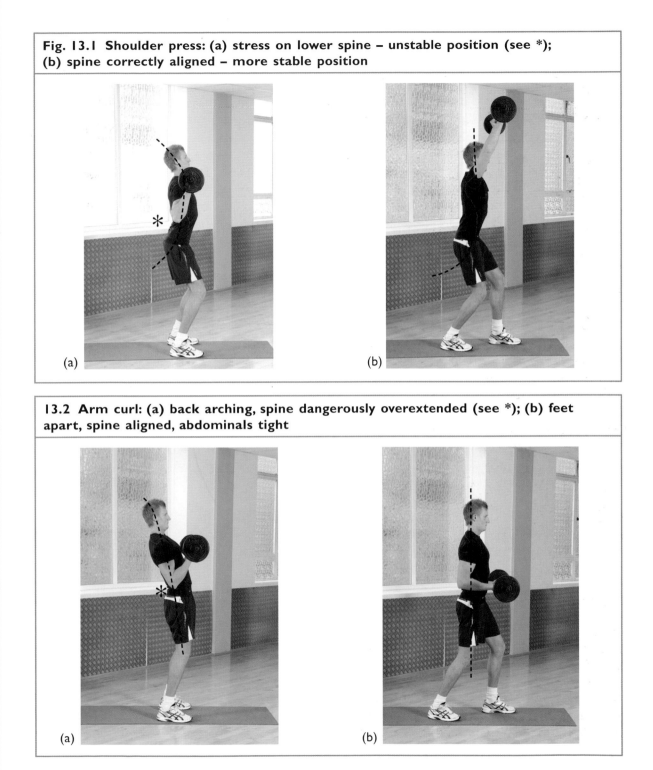

Fig. 13.1 Shoulder press: (a) stress on lower spine – unstable position (see *); (b) spine correctly aligned – more stable position

(a)   (b)

13.2 Arm curl: (a) back arching, spine dangerously overextended (see *); (b) feet apart, spine aligned, abdominals tight

(a)   (b)

In fig. 13.3, the athlete is performing a squat exercise. There are a number of errors in technique here, which are making the exercise quite dangerous to the spine. Firstly, the pelvis has tipped right forwards, allowing the abdominal muscles to lengthen and protrude. This increases the lumbar curve and fails to stabilise the spine. In addition, the knees are not bent sufficiently to lower the weight. Instead the athlete has tipped the trunk forwards on the hip and allowed the spine to move forwards of the ideal posture line. The weight has been pulled forwards, and the leverage (measured as the distance between the weight and the posture line) has increased dramatically.

By applying core stability and posture control principles, the exercise has been modified in fig. 13.3b. The athlete has corrected his posture by bending the knees more (the ankles are raised on a block). This has lowered the weight while keeping the spine and weight close to the posture line. The pelvis is level and the abdominal muscles have been pulled tight by performing the abdominal hollowing action. The spine is therefore more stable and less likely to be injured through excessive joint movement.

Fig. 13.3 Squat exercise: (a) pelvis tipped forwards, increased lumbar curvature, knees not bent, dangerously increased leverage; (b) increased bend in the knees (ankles can be raised on block), pelvis level, spine more stable

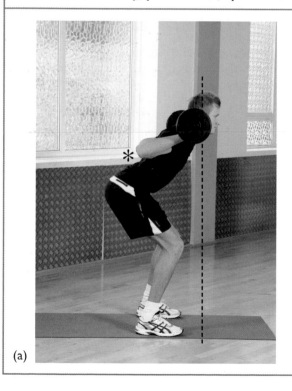
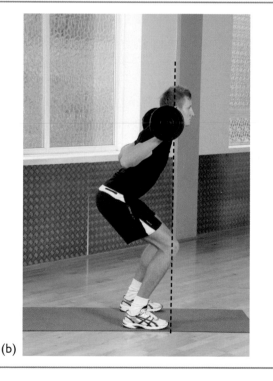

(a)

(b)

Abdominal exercise with weights

Ex 64 Side bend using low pulley

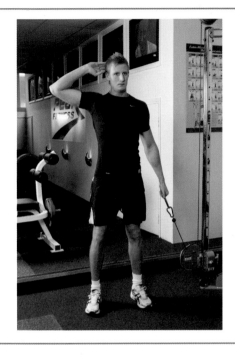 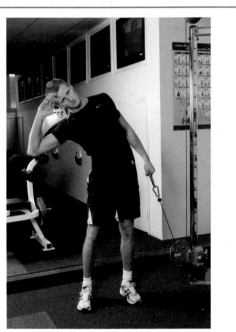

Starting position

Begin standing side-on to a pulley machine. Your feet should be shoulder-width apart and facing forwards. Grip the handle of a low pulley unit in your left hand, taking up any slack in the machine cord. Maintain an optimal posture.

Action

Side-bend your trunk to the right, reaching down the side of your right leg to try to touch the outside of your knee. Pause and then slowly lower the weight to stand upright again.

Points to note

Make sure that you do not lean forwards or backwards as you perform the side-bend. Keep your shoulders and hips square throughout the movement, and do not allow your knees to bend.

Training tip

Focus your attention on the side of your trunk just above the hip. Do not swing the action; bend under control.

Ex 65 Side bend using dumbbell

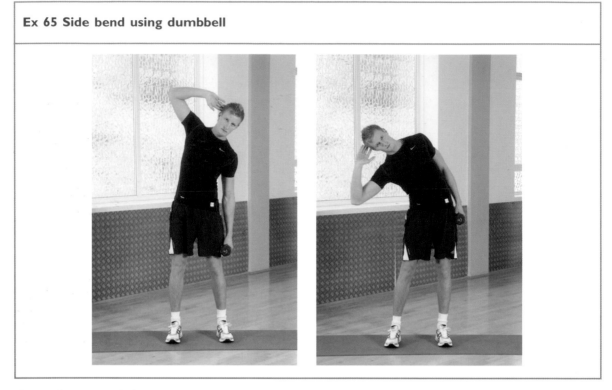

Starting position

Begin standing holding a dumbbell in your left hand. Your feet should be shoulder-width apart and facing forwards. Place your right hand behind your head.

Action

Slowly side-bend your trunk to the left, reaching down the side of your left leg to try to touch the outside of your knee. Pause and then side-bend to the right pulling the dumbbell up to hip level. Once you have finished your set, repeat the action with the dumbbell in your right hand.

Points to note

Make sure that you do not lean forwards or backwards as you perform the side-bend. As you reach downwards, control the descent of the dumbbell, don't allow it to pull you quickly.

Training tip

As you lower the dumbbell your sideflexor muscles of the opposite side of the body (contralateral) are working eccentrically, as you lift they work concentrically. Note: If you use a dumbbell in each hand, the weight of one lowering assists the other to lift and they effectively cancel each other out.

Ex 66 Knee rolling

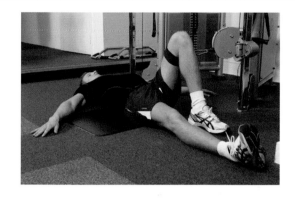 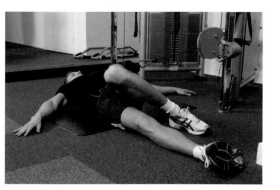

Starting position

Begin lying on your back with one knee bent, the other leg straight. Either attach a sling from a low pulley machine around your bent knee or, if you are working with a partner, use a resistance band. Place your arms out in a 'T' shape to aid stability.

Action

Perform a knee rolling action, lowering your bent knee to the ground away from the pulley or band. As you do this, the weight will lift or the band stretch. Pause and then bring your knee back to the upright position by lowering the weight or releasing the band.

Points to note

Control the movement; do not allow the weight or band to pull you. Once you have performed ten repetitions to one side, change your position to face the other way and perform ten repetitions to this side.

Training tip

If you find the sling from the weight pulley or the band digs into your knee, wrap a towel around your knee beneath the sling/band before you start.

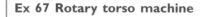

Ex 67 Rotary torso machine

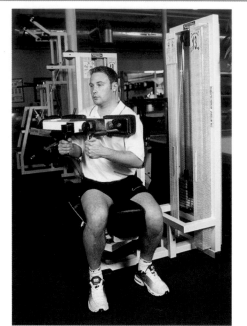 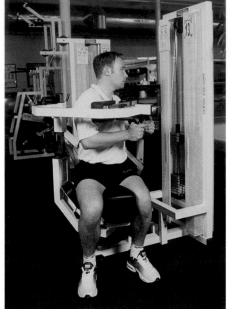

Starting position

Sit on the machine with your knees blocked against the pads. Rest your forearms on the chest bar and grip the handles. Adjust the range of motion limiter so that it allows you to fully twist your spine but not to overstretch it.

Action

Twist to the right then the left, lifting the weight as you do so. Make sure you control the movement in each direction; do not allow the machine to 'run away with you'.

Points to note

The rotary torso action is important as it works the oblique abdominal muscles which are essential to maintain a controlled movement of the spine. However, the range of motion limiter must be set correctly to avoid the risk of the machine twisting you too far. For this reason, set the limiter to stop the machine movement just short of your full degree of spinal twist (full range motion). In this way you will avoid the possibility of overstretching.

Training tip

It is common to be able to move in one direction more easily than the other. This simply represents unequal muscle development (muscular asymmetry) and will correct itself over time.

Ex 68 Abdominal curl machine

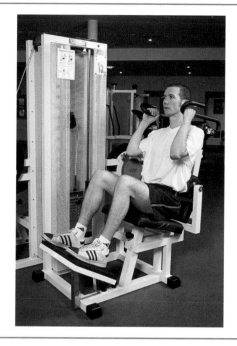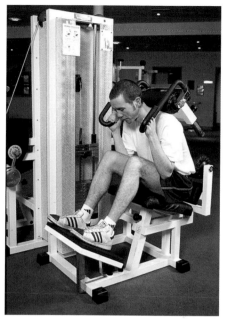

Starting position

Sit on the machine, adjusting the seat height and pads for comfort.

Action

Bend (flex) your trunk reaching your head towards your knees, in a curling action. Hold the inner position and then return.

Points to note

This movement should be a curling action, keeping the lower spine on the seatback and drawing the ribcage down to the pelvis. This will fully tighten (shorten) the muscle. If you simply lean forwards, allowing your lower spine to leave the seatback, the additional movement has occurred at the hip and not the spine.

Training tip

Try to imagine pressing your nose towards your tummy button (*umbilicus*) rather than towards your knees.

Ex 69 Back extension machine

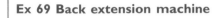

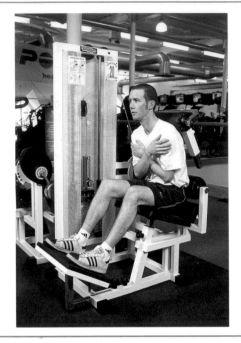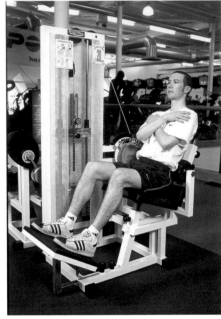

Starting position

Adjust the seat and roller of the back extensor machine for comfort, and fasten the seat belt to hold your pelvis against the machine. Cross your arms across your chest.

Action

Tighten your abdominal muscles and push backwards to lift the weight. Hold the extended position and then lower the weight under careful control.

Points to note

The position of the pivot point of the machine will alter the effect of this exercise. If the pivot is placed at the hip, the action is to tilt the pelvis backwards and extend the spine. With the pivot at the mid-low back (*lumbar spine*), the pelvis will be more difficult to move, but the back will extend further and arch over the machine roller.

Training tip

Press back with the whole of your back, not just your shoulders.

Ex 70 Trunk flexion from high pulley

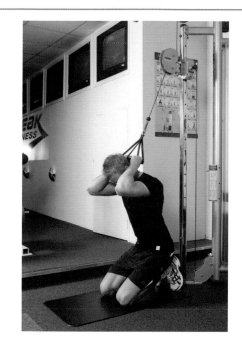 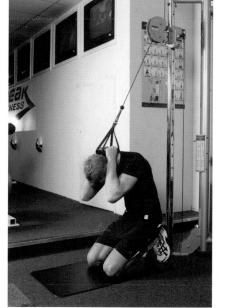

Starting position

Begin sitting astride a bench or kneeling on the floor with your hands behind your neck. Grip the handle of a high pulley unit in both hands, behind your neck.

Action

Flex your trunk, bending it without leaning forwards to lift the weight. Pause and then lower the weight by straightening your trunk again.

Points to note

The action must be one of trunk bending, not bending from the hips.

Training tip

Try to imagine you are aiming to touch your nose to your waist, rather than your nose to your knees. The direction of movement must be down, not forwards.

Ex 71 Side bend from abdominal bench

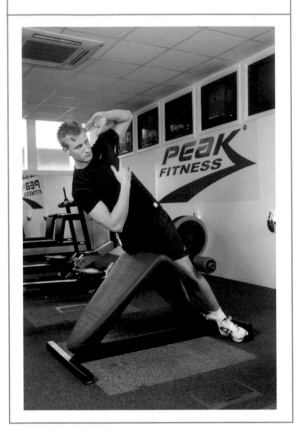

Action

Perform a side-bend action, trying to lift your lower shoulder off the bench. Pause and then slowly lower to the starting position.

Points to note

You may only be able to lift your shoulder by 5–10 cm (2–4 inches). Keep the action strictly to a side bend. Do not lean forwards or backwards.

Training tip

Keep looking forwards as you lift your shoulders, and try to reach your upper hand down towards the side of your upper leg. If you do not have access to an abdominal bench, you can perform this exercise with a training partner holding your feet instead.

Starting position

Lie on your side on a sit-up bench. Hook your feet under the pads, with your upper leg forwards and lower leg back. Fold your lower arm across your chest. Grip your upper shoulder with your hand. Reach along the side of your upper leg with your upper arm.

Ex 72 Spinal extension hold

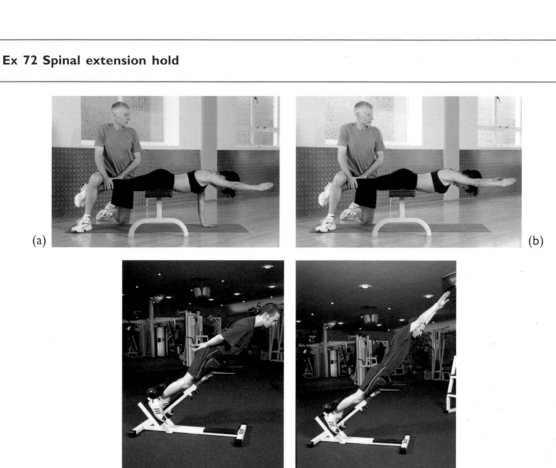

(a)　(b)　(c)　(d)

Starting position

Begin lying across a gym bench in the press-up position, with a training partner holding your feet down (a). This exercise may also be performed on a specific spinal extension frame that has rollers to grip the ankles (c and d).

Action

Perform the abdominal hollowing action to keep your spine in its neutral position. Holding this posture, firstly raise one arm to your side and then both arms. Hold the position and then place your hands back on the ground to rest.

Points to note

You must keep your spine straight throughout this exercise; do not allow it to sag. Do not hold your breath; breathe normally.

Training tip

Try to reach horizontally with the crown of your head and 'lengthen the spine' as you perform the action. Build up the time you can hold the movement until you can hold the correct body position for 30 seconds.

Ex 73 Knee raise hanging

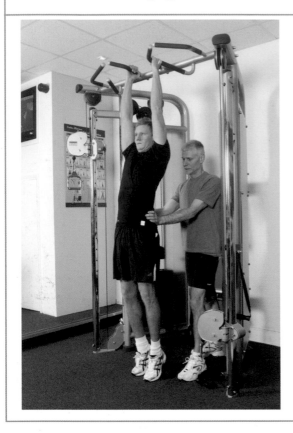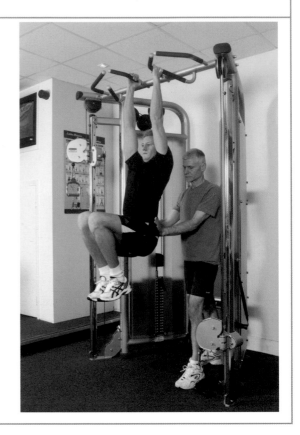

Starting position

Hold onto a chinning bar with your knees bent, feet resting on a bench or the floor.

Action

Bend firstly your knees and hips to bring your legs towards your chest and then bend (flex) your trunk, pulling your tummy button in. Hold the inner position and then lower under control.

Points to note

Try to limit body swing with this movement. Stop after each repetition and rest your feet on the floor or a gym bench.

Training tip

You may also work with a training partner when using this exercise. Ask your partner to stand behind you to prevent you from swinging your body backwards.

Ex 74 Knee raise from frame

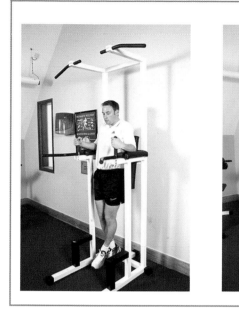 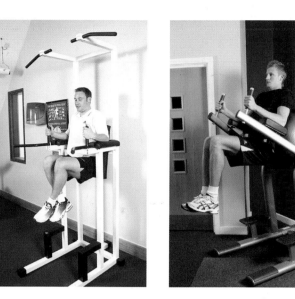

Starting position

Place your forearms on the machine pads and hold onto the handles. Your feet should rest on a gym bench, the floor or the machine footrests.

Action

Bend firstly your knees and hips to bring your legs towards your chest and finally bend (flex) your trunk, pulling your tummy button in. Hold the inner position and then lower under control.

Points to note

This action is the same as exercise 73: knee raise hanging (page 158), but now the need for grip strength, in holding a chinning bar, is removed. However, the action can stress the shoulders if they are allowed to raise up too far.

Training tip

Try to maintain the distance between your shoulders and ears throughout the action, lengthening your spine and 'sitting tall' on the frame. Some machines have a gym ball backrest (*see* photo far right) which makes the exercise harder by introducing an element of balance.

Exercise to music

Core stability principles can be applied to exercise to music (ETM) classes of various types. The aim is to maintain an optimal posture, especially when fatigue sets in at the end of the class, and to control pelvic angulation when performing other exercises.

During step aerobics for example, there is a tendency to allow the pelvis to tilt sideways when taking weight on to the stepping foot (*see* fig. 13.4a). This occurs because the hip muscles and abdominal muscles at the side allow the pelvis to sag. As you take your weight onto your foot, lengthen the spine and stand tall. Keep your pelvis level and tighten your abdominal muscles. Also, ensure that your knee is correctly positioned over the centre of your foot to avoid both knee strain and the faulty knee position pulling the pelvis out of alignment.

Many of the trunk exercises used in ETM classes are performed to very high repetitions. As fatigue sets in there is a tendency for the quality of exercise technique to suffer. Make sure that you are aware of the angle of your pelvis throughout the exercise bout. Do not allow your spine to extend excessively or maintain a flexed posture for any length of time. Try to keep your pelvis in its neutral position.

Keypoint

As fatigue sets in, pay extra attention to your body alignment – failing to do so could cause injury.

Fig. 13.4 Posture during step aerobics: (a) incorrect – pelvis dips, spine leans over, knees have come together; (b) correct – pelvis level, spine lengthened, knees turned out slightly

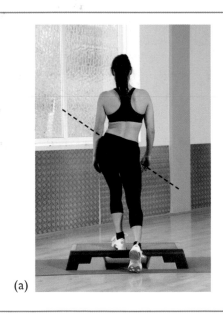

(a)

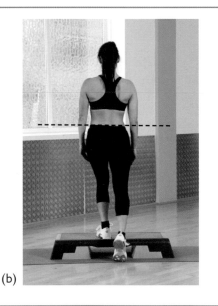

(b)

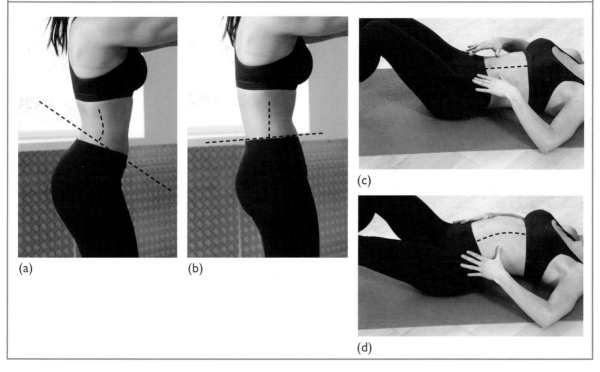

Fig. 13.5 Avoiding hyperextension of the lumber spine in standing: (a) correct position – abdominals pulled in (hollowed), spine neutral; (b) incorrect position – abdominals overtight, pelvis tilted backwards, and lumber spine and lying right; (c) correct; (d) incorrect

Abdominal hollowing is often required to maintain alignment of the spine and pelvis and avoid a 'hollow back' posture (hyperextension stress). In leg lifting exercises, as the leg reaches its maximum angle of extension, the pelvis will tilt and the lower spine hollow unless the abdominal muscles are first tightened. Abdominal hollowing should be performed before the leg is lifted to provide stability to the pelvis and lower spine (*see* fig. 13.5a). Failure to hollow will increase the apparent range of movement of the hip (*see* fig. 13.5b) but the new movement is actually only occurring at the spine.

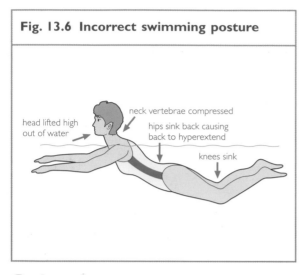

Fig. 13.6 Incorrect swimming posture

head lifted high out of water

neck vertebrae compressed

hips sink back causing back to hyperextend

knees sink

Swimming

Swimming is traditionally seen as a good exercise after a bout of back pain (*see* chapter 15). This is because the body is supported by the water and the jarring which often occurs in exercises on hard floors is avoided. However, failure to maintain a neutral position of the spine can still place considerable stress on the back (*see* fig. 13.6). If breaststroke is used, for example – a style which allows the head to come high above the water surface and the hips to sink – it places stress on both the neck and lower back. Raising the head above the water is a little like standing and looking up at the ceiling for a long time; the neck vertebrae are compressed, especially those of the upper neck. When this happens, the blood flow to the brain is actually reduced and headaches can occur. Always try to breathe out under water when swimming breaststroke so that the head position is lower and the stress to the neck tissues is reduced.

If the hips are allowed to sink, there is more resistance offered by the body. The result is that you have to work harder, and the lower spine is often hyperextended. The abdominal muscles are allowed to relax and lengthen ('ballooning')

and the pelvis tips forward. Again, the vertebrae are compressed, causing inflammation and pain. The answer is to tighten the abdominal muscles slightly to increase core stability and to swim with the body in a more horizontal position.

Abdominal training for speed and power

Many movements in sport are performed rapidly, requiring power and speed. To be specific (*see* chapter 3 for an explanation of training specificity), the abdominal muscles must be trained to match this power requirement. Because these exercises move the spine quickly, they could be potentially dangerous if performed incorrectly. **To lessen the likelihood of injury, you must be able to perform all the exercises correctly for at least ten repetitions using slow movement before you attempt rapid sport-specific actions.**

Rapid actions develop speed; rapid actions performed using weight resistance develop power. Each movement should be performed in a specific sequence to build up intensity gradually. Initially the movements should be slow and controlled until the exercise technique is perfected. Later, the speed of movement is gradually built up without resistance. Only when the action can be performed rapidly, but in a precise, controlled fashion, should resistance be added. Resistance can increase when the exercises no longer feel challenging. Only light resistances should be used as heavy weights will slow the movement and reduce the training effect on power and speed.

Ex 75 Medicine ball curl-up

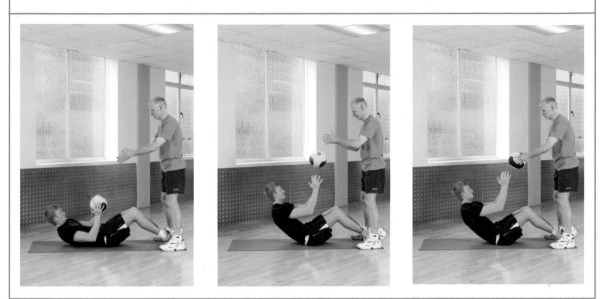

This development of the trunk curl works for explosive power in all of the abdominal muscles. It is especially useful for sports such as gymnastics, where lifting the body is performed at speed.

Do not attempt this exercise until you can perform ten repetitions of exercise 36: trunk curl (page 117), comfortably.

Starting position

Begin the exercise lying on your back on a mat with your knees bent, feet flat but not fixed. Your feet and knees should be spaced wide apart – 50 cm (20 inches). Your training partner should be in the same position (or standing), with their feet about 15–20 cm (6–8 inches) away from yours. If you increase the distance between you to 35–50 cm (14–20 inches) the exercise becomes even harder.

Action

Perform the trunk curl (exercise 36, page 117), and then repeat it using a light, 3 kg (6 lb) medicine ball. As you curl forwards, throw the ball between your knees to your partner, who catches it and throws it back again. Catch the ball in the high position of the exercise and then lower yourself to the floor.

Points to note

Make sure you keep your chin tucked in during this exercise. Do not allow your chin to poke forwards as this will stress the neck considerably.

Training tip

Make sure you keep control of the movement. Do not allow the speed to 'intoxicate you'. Never sacrifice technique for speed, but maintain your alignment throughout the action.

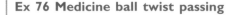

Ex 76 Medicine ball twist passing

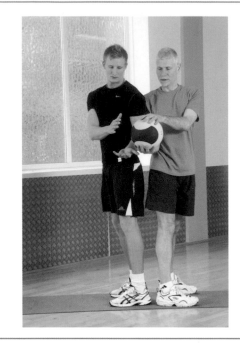 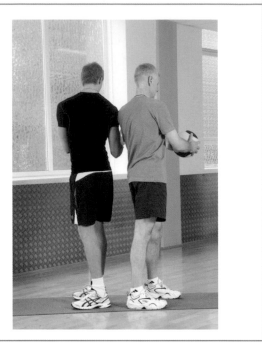

This is useful for building the speed and power of the trunk rotators in combat sports such as judo and wrestling, and also for sports involving rotational movements of the body in space – such as gymnastics, trampolining and board diving.

Starting position

Begin standing back-to-back with a training partner, about 25 cm (10 inches) apart. You should both have your feet shoulder-width apart, standing tall, holding your abdominal muscles in tight.

Action

Hold a medicine ball in both hands and twist round to the right. Your partner twists to the left, takes the medicine ball and then passes it back to you to their right. The movement should be continuous, like two cog wheels working together.

Points to note

Make sure you do not lean back as the movement speeds up.

Training tips

To increase the overload of the exercise stand further apart and throw the medicine ball, using the power of the trunk-twisting action to propel it rather than the arms. Keep the elbows tucked into your sides throughout the movement to reduce the work from the shoulders. If you find this exercise very hard, build the strength of your trunk rotator muscles using exercise 67 for 3-4 weeks beforehand.

Ex 77 Overhead throw-in

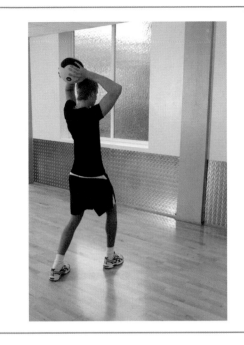 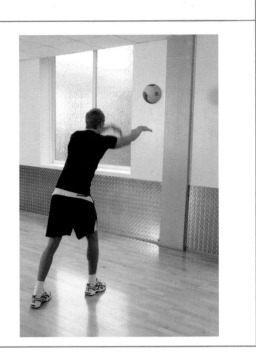

This is useful for building control against forces which tend to press the spine backwards into extension – for instance, in contact and combat sports. This movement is similar to a soccer throw-in.

Starting position

Stand facing a wall with one foot in front of the other. Hold a 3 kg (6 lb) medicine ball in both hands.

Action

Lift the ball overhead and extend the spine, keeping the abdominal muscles tight. Straighten and then slightly flex the spine to throw the ball at the wall. As the ball bounces off, catch it, and control its descent by slightly arching the spine again. Repeat the action.

Points to note

This exercise makes the abdominal muscles work hard to hold the spine stable and prevent it overextending as the ball is thrown and caught. However, excessive movement of the lower spine must be avoided. Be cautious not to overextend the spine when the ball is overhead. The movement should feel comfortable at all times.

Training tip

As the ball bounces off the walls and you catch it, make sure you control it and avoid being pushed into spinal hyperextension. If you find your spine bending too much, throw the ball lower and place your feet further apart.

Ex 78 Punch bag side bend

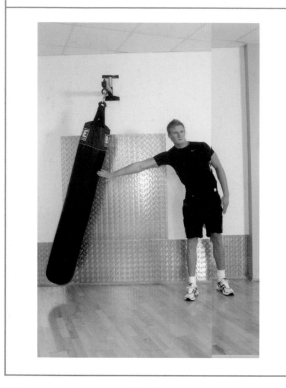

This exercise is useful for building the trunk side flexors both for power movements (gymnastics and trampolining etc.) and to resist blows (contact and combat sports).

Starting position

Begin the exercise standing side-on to a punch bag. Your feet should be shoulder-width apart, and your right arm should be straightened sideways to just touch the punch bag.

Action

Tighten your abdominal muscles slightly and stand tall. Keep your arm straight, and side-bend to the right to push the punch bag. As the bag swings back, control your return to an upright body position. Perform ten repetitions and then turn around so that your left arm touches the punch bag and you side-bend to the left.

Points to note

Make sure you move with the rhythm of the bag, decelerating it as it swings towards you and accelerating it as you push it away.

Training tip

Begin the exercise slowly, with small range movements. Gradually build up the range of motion and speed individually, and then combine the two.

Ex 79 Lunge and reach

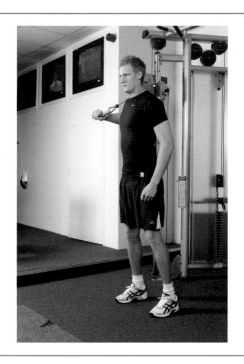 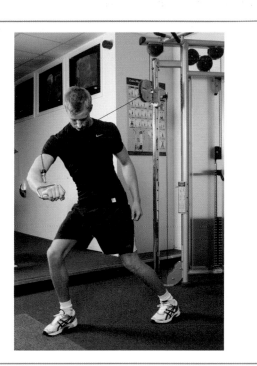

Starting position

Begin standing with your back towards a cable pulley positioned above head height. Hold the 'D' ring of the machine in your right hand and stand with your feet shoulder-width apart.

Action

Step into a lunge position with your right leg and at the same time pull the cable down and across your body to the left. Perform five repetitions then repeat the exercise on the other side of the body, holding the 'D' ring in your left hand and stepping with the left leg.

Points to note

This action combines trunk bending (flexion) and twisting (rotation) while maintaining an upright optimal posture.

Training tip

To begin, limit your movement range. Step forwards by half a metre and reach your hand to waist level only. With practice you can increase the movement range stepping further (1 metre) and reaching lower (to knee or shin level).

Ex 80 Woodchop

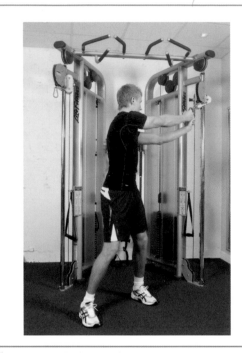
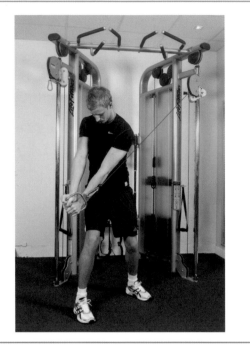

Starting position

Begin standing with your right side facing a cable pulley positioned above head height. Reach to the right and grasp the 'D' ring of the machine in both hands. Stand with your feet 1½ times shoulder-width apart.

Action

Perform a side lunge, taking your weight onto your left leg and, at the same time, reach down to a point in front of your right knee. Perform five repetitions moving to the right and then stand the other way around to perform five repetitions to the left.

Points to note

This action combines trunk bending (flexion), side-bending (lateral flexion) and twisting (rotation) while maintaining an upright optimal posture.

Training tip

To begin, limit your movement range. Take up a shorter lunge position (shoulder width) and pull down to waist level only. With practice you can increase the movement range, widening and deepening the lunge and reaching lower.

Ex 81 Kettlebell snatch lift

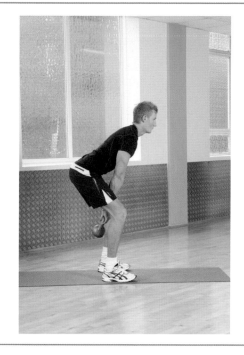 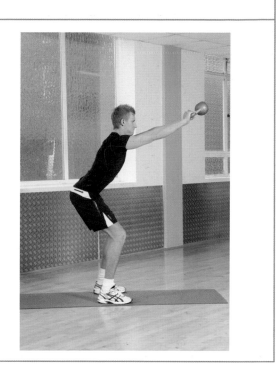

Starting position

Begin in a half-squat position with feet slightly wider than hip-width apart and feet turned out by 10 degrees. Hold a kettlebell between your legs at shin level in both hands. Keep your abdominal muscles tightened and your spine correctly aligned.

Action

Straighten your legs and at the same time reach overhead with your straight arms. Pause in this upper position and then lower the straight arms and bend the knees to position the kettlebell at shin level once more.

Points to note

The action must be to perform the arm lift and stand-up action at the same time. Do not stand up and then lift the arms.

Training tip

If you find the action too intense, begin by placing the kettlebell on a low stool (step bench placed sideways between the legs) and lift from knee height instead.

Ex 82 Kettlebell get up

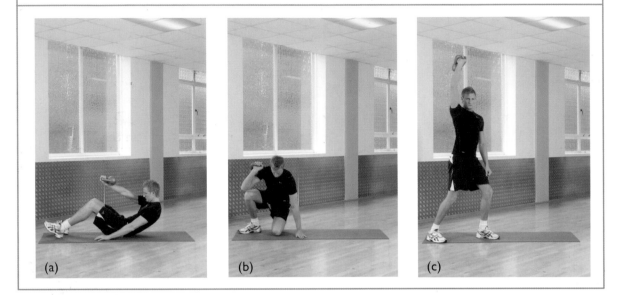

(a)   (b)   (c)

Starting position

Begin sitting on the floor with your knees bent and feet flat. Hold a kettlebell in your right hand and press it overhead, locking the arm (a).

Action

Keeping your right arm locked and overhead all the time, roll onto your left side placing your left hand onto the floor to take up a half-kneeling position (b). Bring your right foot forwards into a lunge position and push up into standing (c). Perform five repetitions holding the kettlebell in your right hand and rolling to the left, five holding it in the left hand and rolling to the right.

Points to note

This is a complex exercise involving core stability and coordination. Use a light kettlebell (4 kg) to begin with until you can perform the action smoothly.

Training tip

If you find the coordination difficult, split the movement into two phases: phase one, turning into the half-kneeling position for three repetitions; phase two, begin in half-kneeling and move to standing for three repetitions. Rest, and then put both phases together to perform the whole kettlebell get up exercise.

ABDOMINAL TRAINING AND PREGNANCY

14

In this chapter we look at abdominal training both during pregnancy and after childbirth. Abdominal training is essential in both instances, but we need to understand a little about what the body goes through during pregnancy and childbirth and discuss a few precautions. As well as your GP and midwife, two professionals may be of help to you during this stage of your life – a physiotherapist specialising in women's health, and a personal trainer who offers advice on postnatal fitness.

Before we focus on the abdominal muscles, let's take a brief look at the general changes that your body goes through during pregnancy.

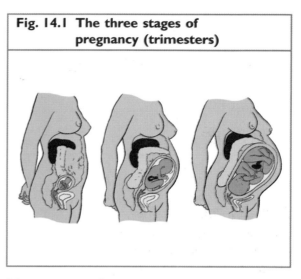

Fig. 14.1 The three stages of pregnancy (trimesters)

Body changes during pregnancy

Your pregnancy can be divided into three phases, called *trimesters*, each of approximately three months duration. The first trimester is from conception to week 12, the second from week 12 to week 28, and the third from week 28 to childbirth. During this time, your body goes through some remarkable changes. Your uterus grows from being about the size of a tennis ball to somewhere near the size of a football, and the amount of blood in your body (blood volume) increases by about 40 per cent. This is reflected by an increase in bodyweight. This is usually around 10 to 12 kg (22–26 lb), but may be less if you are normally overweight and more if you are quite lean.

Hormone changes

You will go through many hormone changes during pregnancy. Progesterone and oestrogen levels increase, stopping your menstrual cycle, and prolactin levels instigate changes in your breasts. Your breasts may be tender during the first trimester especially, as they begin to change. Their weight and shape alters as fat- and milk-producing tissue is formed. Have your bra size measured regularly and wear a supporting bra (but not an underwired bra, as it can restrict natural movement).

> **Keypoint**
>
> You bra size will increase throughout pregnancy, be sure to get professionally measured a number of times.

Pregnancy hormones will also have an affect on your bladder and it is quite normal to need to go to the toilet more often. Don't try to compensate for this by cutting down on fluids, however, because you will need additional fluids during exercise. You may also find that you retain more fluids and notice swelling in your legs, ankles and feet. Exercise will help with this by increasing circulation and fluid movement. Also, try not to stand for long periods, and elevate your legs whenever possible.

At the beginning of pregnancy, as your hormones begin to change, your blood vessels become more elastic and relax (vasodilation). Because at this early stage you have the same amount of circulating blood, there is actually too little to fill the blood vessels (vascular underfill). The result of these changes is that you may feel dizzy and faint, especially when getting up from the floor or a gym bench. During this stage, try to avoid exercises which involve prolonged standing and, when you get up from floor work, do so in stages. Turn onto your side, wait a few seconds, then push up onto your hands and knees and wait. Bring one foot through so you kneel on one knee, and finally move to standing slowly, again taking a few seconds to 'get your bearings' (*see* exercise 83, opposite).

> **Keypoint**
>
> Circulation changes, particularly in the first trimester, may leave you feeling lightheaded when you change body position.

Relaxin hormone

From the point of view of abdominal exercise, it is the hormone *relaxin* which is the most important. This hormone is normally produced in your ovaries and breasts, but during pregnancy additional amounts come from the placenta and the lining of your uterus (endometrium). It is released from about week two in pregnancy and its effects can stay in your body for up to five months after childbirth. During pregnancy the relaxin hormone softens connective tissue within the body by increasing the amount of water taken up by the collagen fibres within this tissue. The result of this softening is to allow the joints of the pelvis (sacrociliac at the back and pubis at the front) to 'give' a little so that the pelvis can expand to allow childbirth. The softening does not just affect the pelvic joints, however, but all of the joints in the body. For this reason you must be cautious with high-impact activities and intense stretching.

> **Keypoint**
>
> Joints soften during pregnancy and remain soft for up to five months after childbirth. Be cautious about exercises which place high stress levels on your joints.

Abdominal and pelvic muscles during pregnancy

We have seen that your uterus is increasing in size throughout pregnancy. This results in changes to your abdominal cavity or 'balloon' (*see* fig. 14.2a, page 174). The weight of the uterus is supported at the bottom of the cavity by the ligaments and muscles making up your pelvic floor (*see* fig. 14.2b). The uterus 'hangs' within the pelvis supported by the *round ligaments* positioned at either side attached to the front of the pelvis, and the *broad ligament* attached from the uterine sac to the lumbar spine. The increasing size and weight of the uterus stretches the ligaments and may give discomfort in the lower abdomen. This can be eased by keeping the pelvic floor muscles strong and practising core stability exercises.

Ex 83 Moving from lying to standing

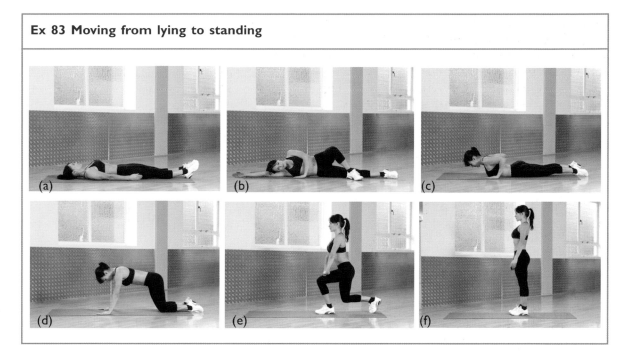

Starting position

Begin lying on your back on a mat.

Action

Keeping your body horizontal (do not sit up) turn onto your right side (b), and then onto your front (c). Push with your arms to press your hips backwards (d), bending your knees to come up to a kneeling position (four point kneeling, hands and knees on the ground). Draw your right foot and leg forwards (e) and place your right foot flat on the floor (half kneeling, one knee on the ground). Place both hands on top of your right knee and press downwards on the knee to propel yourself to standing. Bring your feet together (f).

Points to note

As you bring your right foot forwards and press onto your knee, try to keep your shin bone (tibia) vertical with a 90 degree angle at your knee. This will position the force of your push along the shin bone and give you better leverage to push into standing.

Training tip

If you feel dizzy moving from lying to standing, pause at each position change and allow your breathing to settle before moving onto the next position.

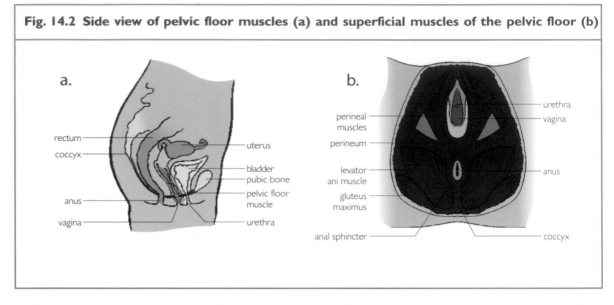

Fig. 14.2 Side view of pelvic floor muscles (a) and superficial muscles of the pelvic floor (b)

The pelvic floor muscles are called the *levator ani* and are actually three small pairs of muscles. They form a muscular sling which contains the anus, vagina, and urethra. The muscles, like any others in the body, are able to provide both low grade tone over a period of time (endurance) and sudden high tone of short duration (power and speed). The former is required to offer continual support of the pelvic contents throughout the day, the latter gives extra support when you cough or sneeze. It is important to re-develop both endurance and speed of contraction following childbirth to prevent incontinence.

Pelvic floor re-education

It is important to re-educate your pelvic floor even if you have had a caesarean section (c-section). With a c-section the pelvic floor muscles have not been stretched as they would with a natural childbirth, but they have supported your baby for nine months and relaxin hormone has made them more elastic. In natural childbirth the pelvic floor has been stretched and may have been damaged. You will

usually have had a tear at the vaginal opening, and may have had an episiotomy (surgical incision) and stitches. Do not forget about your pelvic floor! Here is a frightening statistic to motivate you to use the exercises below: one in four women (that's right, a quarter of the female population) over the age of 40 suffers from some form of incontinence. Much of this is preventable.

Firstly, let's find out how strong your pelvic floor is. Clinically a physiotherapist will assess this using palpation (touching) and a machine called a perineometer (a type of pressure gauge that is inserted into the vagina). You can get some idea of the strength of your pelvic floor muscles next time you go to the toilet. When you pass water, try to stop your urine stream mid-flow. If you are able to do this and hold it for 2–3 seconds without any dribbling, your pelvic floor is quite strong. Use this as a test, but do not keep doing it as stopping the urine flow in this way repeatedly can increase the chance of getting a bladder infection.

Now, lets look at three pelvic floor exercises which you can use regularly.

Ex 84 Pelvic floor contraction standing

Starting position

Begin standing with your feet hip-width apart, arms by your sides. Breathe normally; do not hold your breath during the exercise.

Action

Focus your attention on the area between your legs. Without moving or squeezing your legs together, imagine that you are pulling your perineal area (crotch) upwards. Hold the upward position and then release.

Points to note

Initially you may not notice anything happening. Persevere, however, because by imagining the movement (visualisation) the nervous impulses going to these muscles will actually increase. Eventually you will feel a small flicker of contraction, but don't be disappointed if it takes five sessions of trying before anything happens.

Training tip

Close your eyes and imagine your pelvic floor as a piece of cloth. As you contract, think of lifting the cloth up inside your vagina slightly.

Ex 85 Pelvic floor contraction sitting

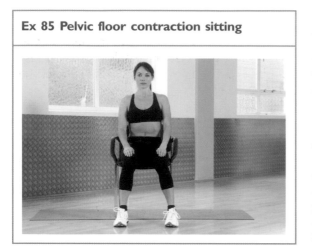

Starting position

Sit on a firm dining chair with your feet hip-width apart. Sit up tall; do not slouch.

Action

Focus your attention on your sitting bones (ischial tuberosities) and tighten your pelvic floor muscles, imagining that you are pulling your sitting bones together. Next, focus your attention on your pubic bone and tailbone (coccyx) and, as you contract your pelvic floor, imagine that you are pulling these two bones together. Finally, contract your pelvic floor and imagine that you are pulling all four points (both sitting bones, tailbone and pubis) together.

Points to note

When focussing on the ischial tuberosities you are reducing the side-to-side (lateral) distance of the pelvic floor. By focussing on the tailbone and pubis you are reducing the front-to-back (*antero-posterior*) distance.

Training tip

Some people find the imagery of a fairground claw crane (candy grabber) useful. Imagine the four points are the ends of the grabber and, as you contract your pelvic floor, you are closing the claw and picking something up.

Ex 86 Pelvic floor pulsing

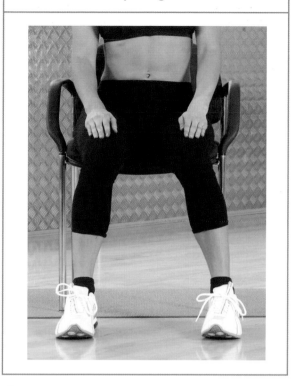

Action

Focus your attention on your perineum and tighten your pelvic floor muscles, pulling them in and up. Tighten quickly, and then relax the muscles quickly.

Points to note

The aim of this exercise is to switch the muscles on and off rapidly to train muscle reaction time. Perform this exercise after you have mastered exercise 84 (page 175) and have a confident pelvic floor contraction.

Training tip

You may find the first repetition of this exercise quite weak, but as you continue each contraction should increase in intensity.

Starting position

Sit on a firm dining chair with your feet hip-width apart. Sit up tall; do not slouch.

Abdominal muscles and childbirth

During pregnancy the abdominal muscles have to stretch to accommodate your growing baby. The muscles are able to stretch lengthways quite substantially, but their ability to stretch sideways is limited. The sideways increase in space is brought about by the splitting of tissue which joins the two neighbouring central abdominal muscles (rectus abdominis on each side – *see* fig. 14.3). The split is called a *diastasis* and this is usually focussed around the tummy button (umbilicus) extending upwards and downwards from this point. The width of the diastasis (the inter-recti distance) can be measured using ultrasound scanning. Maximum widths are described as no greater than 0.9 cm midway between the pubis and umbilicus, 2.7 cm just above the umbilicus and 1.0 cm midway between the umbilicus and bottom of the breast bone (xyphoid). A diastasis exceeding these measurements may require surgical repair.

The size of the diastasis is dependent on a number of factors. Mothers who have a narrow pelvis or a large baby (over 9 lb) are likely to have a larger diastasis, as are those who have twins or triplets. If a mother has been inactive during her pregnancy or has not toned up the abdominal muscles following a previous pregnancy, again the diastasis may be larger.

During pregnancy and following childbirth, core stability and pelvic tilting actions are both important to reduce the strain on the abdominal wall and the spine. Following child birth, the diastasis must be allowed to close before very active abdominal exercises are begun. Abdominal hollowing is particularly useful during the early stages post-childbirth (from three days). The action should be practised regularly throughout the day to re-educate the abdominal muscles. It is often easier to practise

this movement while breast feeding in a sitting or lying position: as a young mum you will have little time available; the feeding period may be the only respite you have.

Pelvic tilting is also important during the first weeks after child birth. The aim now is to correct any exaggeration in the lumbar curve (lordosis) which occurs through a forward-tilted pelvis (*see* fig. 1.15, page 11). Whenever you are standing, you should try to do so without an excessive curve in the lower spine.

The oblique abdominal muscles pull onto the area of the tummy which has split during pregnancy. Forcible contraction of the obliques may therefore slow the closure of the diastasis, so twisting actions against resistance should not be practised until the diastasis has closed to a width of two fingers.

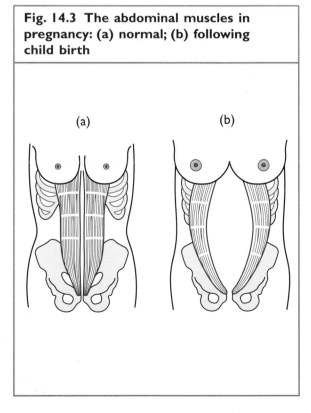

Fig. 14.3 The abdominal muscles in pregnancy: (a) normal; (b) following child birth

(a) (b)

Abdominal muscle re-education following childbirth

For the week following childbirth, two activities are important. Firstly, try to practise pelvic floor contractions regularly throughout the day, and secondly focus on good backcare. Try to build the pelvic floor contractions into your daily routine. Use them when you are standing and cleaning your teeth, waiting for the kettle to boil, sitting at a traffic light, for example, rather than taking separate time out. This way, the actions become more functional as they are used during normally activities rather than separate from them.

In terms of general backcare, try to reduce the amount of spine bending that you do, focusing on bending the knees and not your back. I know it is a familiar adage to 'keep your back straight and bend your knees', but it is really important to prevent stress accumulating on the lower back. If you develop a cough and find coughing painful (especially if you have a caesarian scar) press a large, soft pillow over your abdomen or use the flat of your hands over your scar to support yourself.

When you begin to use abdominal training itself, practise the abdominal hollowing action and pelvic tilting. Begin in kneeling (exercise 14 page 91) because this will probably be the most comfortable position for your low back. Remember to get down into the kneeling position without bending, using exercise 83 (page 173). Once you are confident with the hollowing action, use exercise 16 (page 93) and exercise 18 (page 95) as well. Aim for 5–10 repetitions of each exercise.

Try to build your general fitness with walking/powerwalking before returning to the gym. If you are walking with your baby in a carrier, make sure the straps are adjusted correctly so that your shoulders do not round. Equally, if you are pushing a buggy try to stand

Table 14.1	Example of abdominal training following childbirth
Time from childbirth	Exercise
Week 1	• General backcare and pelvic floor re-education. • Begin abdominal hollowing in sitting, 5 single reps with a 5 second rest between each, 3 times a day. • Begin pelvic tilting, aiming to reduce the depth of your lumbar curve if it is excessive (see fig. 1.15). • Support scars when coughing. • Walking 5–10 minutes practising good posture control.
Week 2/3	• Continue pelvic floor exercise. • Increase walking to 15–20 mins. • Add abdominal hollowing in kneeling, 2 sets of 5 reps, and pelvic tilting in standing, 2 sets of 5 reps. • At end of week 2 add Exercise 24, 5 reps each leg.
Week 4/5	• General gym work to include CV and resistance. • Core stability foundation movements moving onto level one when all exercises are pain free and performed with good technique.

as upright as possible so that you do not get low back pain.

You may find that you have a hollow back (lordotic) posture during pregnancy and following childbirth. Practise pelvic tilting (exercise 11, page 87) to regain control of your lumbopelvic region. When you feel ready, work through the foundation movements and progress to the level one exercises. Also increase your general exercise to include CV work and some resistance training.

Summary

- Relaxin hormone will make your joints less stable and more susceptible to damage from intense stretching.
- It is essential to practise pelvic floor exercises during pregnancy and following childbirth.
- The split in the abdominal muscles which occurs during pregnancy is called a 'diastasis'.
- The diastasis may be larger if you have a narrow pelvis, a large baby or twins, or are overweight.
- The abdominal hollowing exercise can help regain your figure.
- Vigorous abdominal training is dangerous after pregnancy.

ABDOMINAL TRAINING IN THE POOL

15

Water has a number of advantages for any exercise involving the spine. The warmth of water is soothing, making it very useful following back pain. In addition, water will support the body, taking some of the bodyweight off the joints and spine and so will reduce pain. The muscles responsible for maintaining posture need to work less in water as well because your posture is supported by the water itself.

For the elderly, who may have circulatory problems as well as back pain, water has a further advantage. The pressure variation from the bottom of the pool to the surface actually helps the blood to return to the heart from the legs (venous return) and so reduces 'tired legs'. Furthermore, the pressure changes created by the depth of the water assist in the reduction in blood pooling (blue veins in the legs) and swelling around the ankles.

> ### Keypoint
>
> Pressure variation from the bottom of a pool to the top aids venous return, a feature especially important in those individuals with poor circulation in their legs.

Principles of water exercise

Buoyancy

Buoyancy is the degree to which your body will float when it is in water. Your individual buoyancy is determined by your body make-up. Body fat will make you more buoyant, while muscle makes you less. Plump individuals will tend to float, therefore, while those who are skinny are more likely to sink.

The distribution of your body fat is also important. Those with more fat around the waist and lower body (pear shape) will find that their legs float more while leaner individuals find their legs sink. This is why, in general, men float deeper in the water than women. If you do float lower in the water, you may find some of the exercises easier if you use floats.

The depth of the water you are standing in will also affect your buoyancy. The body will float more when it is in deeper water. When the water is waist high, your bodyweight is

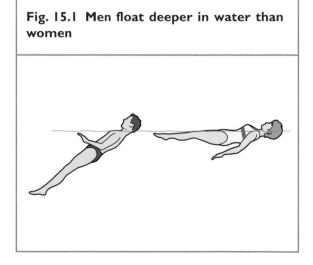

Fig. 15.1 Men float deeper in water than women

actually reduced by about 50 per cent. When the water is up to your shoulders, your body-weight is effectively reduced by 90 per cent, so there is considerably less shock on the joints and spine in deeper water. This is what makes deep water training so effective at maintaining CV fitness without jolting the spine and leg joints. However, because you float more in deeper water, movement can be harder to control, so be cautious.

> ### Keypoint
>
> Buoyancy is related to body density. Thinner and more muscular individuals tend to sink, while those with higher body fat will float.

Buoyancy can be used to support parts of the body, and both to assist and resist movements. In fig. 15.2a, the subject is lying flat in the water, holding on to the siderail of the swimming pool. To enable him to float he has placed a rubber ring around his waist, and a smaller ring around his legs. The rings can be inflated or deflated according to the subject's buoyancy, to allow the body to float either just beneath the surface of the water or deeper. This supported lying position enables a selection of spinal exercises to be performed with the body moving freely in several directions.

In fig. 15.2b, buoyancy is being used for assistance. The subject is performing a knee lift movement, but the legs are too heavy to perform the movement correctly. A ring has been placed around the knees to allow the legs to float partially, in effect making them lighter and assisting the upward action of the legs. In fig. 15.2c, the reverse situation is occurring. The exercise is hip extension, pressing the leg downwards. Now, the buoyancy of the rubber ring tending to lift the leg upwards is acting as a resistance to the downwards movement of the leg.

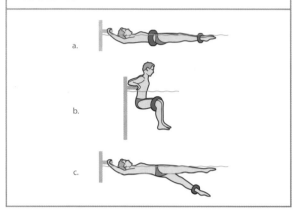

Fig. 15.2 Buoyancy: (a) flotation aids; (b) buoyancy assistance; (c) buoyancy resistance

> ### Keypoint
>
> Buoyancy can be used to assist or resist a movement, and to support a body part during exercise.

Resistance

Resistance is also provided by the movement of an object through water. The greater the amount of water which has to move, and the faster the object moves, the greater the resistance. Placing the hand side-on (*see* fig. 15.3 (2)) and moving it slowly through the water provides a certain resistance to the arm muscles performing the movement. If the hand is turned through 90 degrees so that it faces vertically (*see* fig. 15.3 (1)), it provides considerably more resistance to movement and so the arm muscles must work harder. Speeding up the movement increases the workload still further.

To boost muscle work further we can use apparatus to increase resistance (*see* fig. 15.3 (4 and 5)). Floats placed on their sides and webbed hand gloves are both useful to enhance a water workout.

Fig. 15.3 Using water resistance

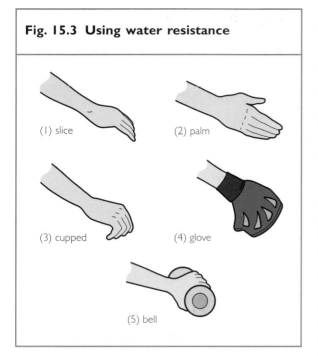

(1) slice

(2) palm

(3) cupped

(4) glove

(5) bell

Other water apparatus is also useful to offer variety in exercises including aquatubes (woggles), steps, plastic dumbbells (*see* fig. 15.3 (5)), and a buoyancy aid for deep water training.

Because fast movements offer greater resistance, rapid limb movements are useful when working on trunk stability. Standing in deep water and pushing a float rapidly forwards and backwards, for example, will tend to displace the trunk. Tightening the abdominal muscles against this displacement will enhance trunk stability.

Safety considerations

Obviously water is a dangerous medium to work in, but these dangers can be considerably reduced by taking sensible precautions. Poor swimmers should never practise water exercises in water above waist height, and they must stay close to the poolside at all times. Young children must be continuously supervised, however strong their swimming may appear.

When using apparatus to float, it is easy to become disorientated, which can lead to panic. For this reason, always exercise with a partner. When one of you is working, the other should be standing by, offering support and encouragement.

Many accidents occur when moving to and from the pool, so *walk* on wet surfaces, don't run. Also, be cautious when getting into and out of the pool, and use the steps rather than jumping or diving in, especially when you are exercising in shallow water.

Keypoint

In water, it's always safety first.

Keypoint

Less streamlined objects offer greater water resistance, and can be used to make an exercise harder.

Water exercises

Ex 87 Trunk side bending

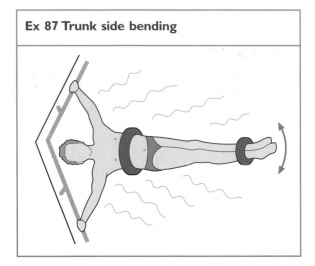

Starting position

Begin the exercise lying on your back in the water, holding on to the siderail of the pool. Choose a wide grip, and keep your arms locked. Ask your training partner to place a rubber ring around your waist, and a smaller (or less inflated) ring around your shins. The rings should be inflated sufficiently to allow your body to float just beneath the surface of the water.

Action

Keep your legs straight and move them from side to side in the water to make your trunk side-flex. Keep the action slow and controlled, and pause as you reach the end point of each sideways movement.

Points to note

Make sure you control the momentum of the movement. Do not allow yourself to be forced into a greater side-bending range of motion than you intended.

Training tip

Begin the exercise slowly with small-range movements. Gradually build up the range of motion and speed individually and then combine the two.

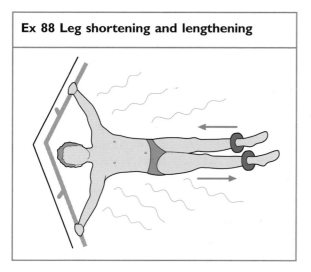

Ex 88 Leg shortening and lengthening

Starting position

Place floats around your ankles, and lie in the water on your back. Grip the siderail of the pool, or lie in the corner of the pool with your arms on each wall.

Action

Keep your body in line, and shorten one leg while lengthening the other, so that your pelvis tilts sideways.

Points to note

Do not allow your spine to bend (flex) or hollow (extend) – instead, isolate the movement to the pelvis.

Training tip

If you find the movement difficult to visualise, have a training partner hold a float at your feet. Watch each foot moving towards and then away from the float.

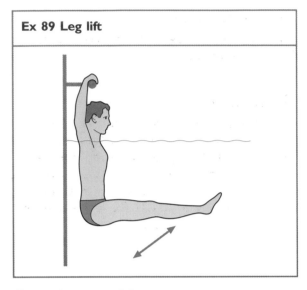

Ex 89 Leg lift

Starting position

Hold on to the siderail above head height. Keep your back flat against the poolside.

Action

Lift and lower your legs, keeping them straight, and tighten your abdominal muscles using the abdominal hollowing procedure.

Points to note

If you find this movement difficult, place a rubber ring around your legs to assist you in the lifting motion.

Training tip

If the movement seems very easy, perform the action more quickly to increase the resistance from the water.

Ex 90 Resisted trunk rotation

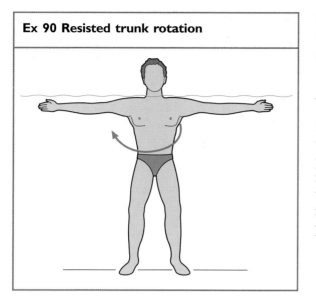

Points to note

Twist round as far as is comfortable, but do not force the movement.

Training tip

If you find the exercise easy, either wear webbed gloves, or hold a float in each hand positioned at 90 degrees to the water surface to increase resistance. Speeding up the movement will also make the exercise harder due to increased water resistance, but make sure that you maintain a good posture.

Starting position

Begin the exercise standing in chest deep water within reach of the poolside. Place your feet shoulder-width apart and stand tall, pulling your tummy in. Stretch your arms out to the side, keeping them just below the surface of the water. Your hands should be flat at 90 degrees to the surface of the water, fingers together.

Action

Twist your trunk firstly to the right and then to the left, without bending forwards or backwards.

Ex 91 Knee twist

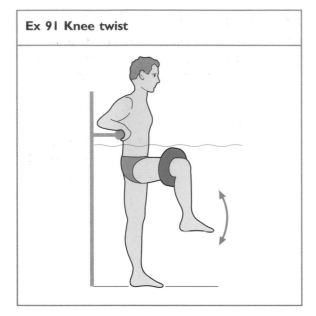

Starting position

Begin the exercise with your back on the poolside, gripping the siderail with both hands. Bend one knee and place a rubber ring around the knee of this leg.

Action

Tighten your abdominal muscles and flatten the small of your back towards the poolside. Keeping the tummy tight, twist the trunk to bring the bent knee across the body. Perform five repetitions to one side, then change legs and perform five repetitions to the other side.

Points to note

Everyone is asymmetrical and it is common to be able to twist further in one direction than the other.

Training tip

Initially, rather than performing a continuous action, twist, pause, and twist back.

Ex 92 Body curl

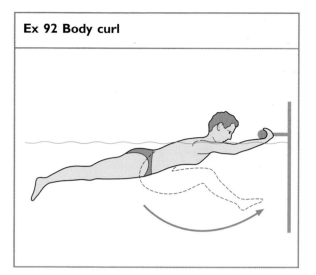

Starting position

Lie on your front, and grip the siderail of the pool.

Action

Bend the legs and trunk to bring your knees towards your chest, and your feet onto the poolside. Pause, and then stretch the body out straight again.

Points to note

The knees begin the movement, followed by the hips and finally the spine. The order is reversed as the legs extend once more.

Training tips

The movement becomes harder if a float is placed around the feet, as buoyancy resists the leg movement under the surface of the water.

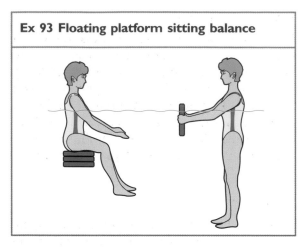

Ex 93 Floating platform sitting balance

Starting position

In shallow water (waist deep or up to lower chest level only) sit on enough floats to allow your body to float in the seated position with the water to the level of your chest.

Action

Tighten (hollow) your abdomen and sit up straight. Have your training partner stand in front of you, feet apart. Your partner holds a float vertically and forces the water against you by pushing with their float, while you try to stay sitting upright. You will have to tighten your abdominal muscles harder to do this.

Points to note

If you find it difficult to maintain balance while sitting on the platform, move into shallower water so that your feet rest on the bottom. Also use fewer floats to ensure that all of your chest is in the water.

Training tip

Once able to maintain your balance, your partner should vary the water current by pushing harder/softer, faster/slower, and from different directions. The aim is to vary the amount of muscle contraction used, to match the changing force of the water being pressed against you.

Ex 94 Aquatube sitting balance

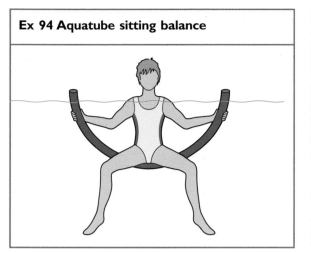

Starting position

Sit on the tube and grasp the two ends in much the same way as a child would on a swing.

Action

Sit upright and abdominal hollow. Hold the position as you balance on the aquatube.

Points to note

Make sure that you select an aquatube which is suitable for your body size. If you are quite heavy or muscular and have a greater tendency to sink, you will need a larger aquatube. If you have quite a lot of bodyfat and float easily, too big an aquatube will cause you to float too high in the water. Select a tube that allows you to float with the water level at your shoulders.

Training tip

If you find the balance of this exercise quite hard, have a training partner stand behind you and steady your hips. If you find the exercise very easy, again use a training partner, but this time have them use a float to push and pull the water around you to challenge your balance.

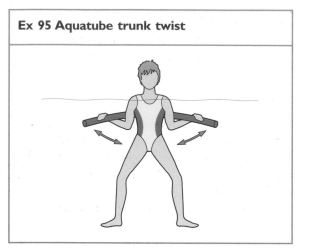

Ex 95 Aquatube trunk twist

Points to note

Twisting more quickly will make the exercise harder as water resistance will increase.

Training tip

Make sure you grip the pool floor firmly with your feet before you start. If you are too high in the water your feet will slide.

Starting position

Begin standing in shoulder-high water with your feet slightly wider than shoulder-width apart, knees slightly bent (soft). Place the aquatube behind your upper back so that it stays in the water throughout the exercise.

Action

Twist to the right then the left, pressing the tube against the resistance of the water.

Ex 96 Aquatube push down

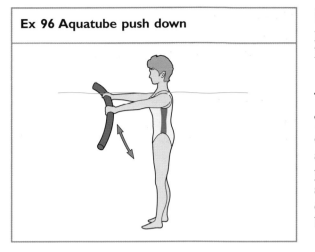

Points to note

Pushing down more quickly makes the exercise harder due to increased water resistance.

Training tip

To increase the work on your abdominals, you can flex the trunk slightly as you push the aquatube downwards. However, make sure that you don't flex so much that you position your shoulders over the top of the tube as this will enable you to press down on the tube with your bodyweight alone.

Starting position

Begin standing in shoulder-high water with your feet slightly wider than shoulder-width apart, knees slightly bent (soft). Hold the aquatube in front of you with your arms shoulder-width apart and straight.

Action

Stabilise your trunk and, keeping your arms straight, push the aquatube downwards towards your thighs. Pause in the lower position and then allow the tube to float up under control, again keeping your arms straight.

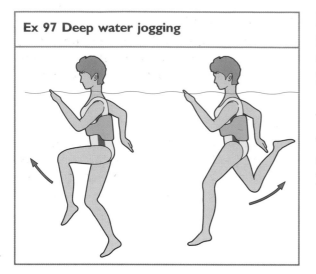

Ex 97 Deep water jogging

Points to note

Make sure you float with the water at the top of your chest. If you are too high in the water, you may angle your trunk forwards into flexion.

Training tip

This action unloads your spine from compression forces and is especially good for regaining your CV fitness following a back injury.

Starting position

Fasten a buoyancy belt around your chest so that you can float with your feet above the floor of the pool. Swim 1.5m away from the side of the pool so that you do not kick the pool wall, but still keep yourself within easy reach if you need support.

Action

Stand tall, and jog in the water reaching your arms forwards and moving your legs in a cycling action. Jog for 2 minutes and then reverse the action, using a backwards movement with your arms and legs.

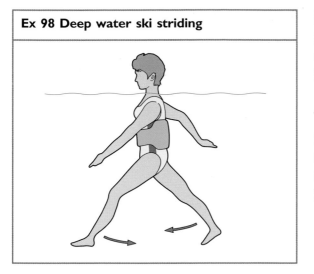

Ex 98 Deep water ski striding

Points to note

Make sure you float with the water around the shoulder area. If you are too high in the water, you may angle your trunk forwards into flexion.

Training tip

Like deep water jogging (exercise 97, page 194) this action unloads your spine from compression forces and is especially good for regaining your CV fitness following a back injury.

Starting position

Fasten a buoyancy belt around your chest so that you can float with your feet above the floor of the pool. Swim 1.5m away from the side of the pool so that you do not kick the pool wall, but still keep yourself within easy reach if you need support.

Action

Stand tall and stride in the water keeping your arms and legs straight. Stride for 3-4 minutes using an even gait, and then perform 1 minute using a longer stride.

ABDOMINAL TRAINING FOLLOWING SURGERY

16

Many people tend to think that after surgery on the abdomen they will always have weakness and a 'floppy tummy'. This is not true. Although a scar is present and the muscles have been affected, it is possible to re-train the abdominal muscles and get full function back in this area.

Surgical operation scars

Following a surgical operation in the abdominal region, you are left with a scar; its size and position will dictate the type and intensity of abdominal training appropriate.

There are many positions for scars and fig. 16.1 shows some of the most common.

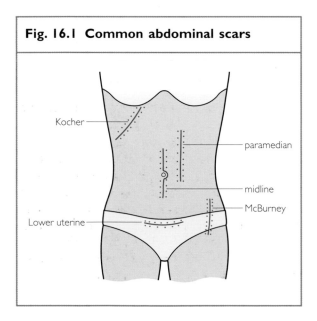

Fig. 16.1 Common abdominal scars

Kocher

paramedian

midline

McBurney

Lower uterine

Essentially an incision is either *vertical*, travelling down the length of the body, *transverse* going across at 90 degrees, or *oblique*, travelling at an angle. The size of the scar will be dependent on the procedure carried out and the structure affected. A lot of surgery is carried out using keyhole procedures; a number of tiny scars are left where the fibre optic camera and small instruments used by the surgeon were passed through.

In most operations a surgeon prefers to cut between (split), rather than through, muscle fibres making healing quicker and stronger. Larger nerves are generally avoided but, because small nerve branches may have been cut during surgery, your scar area may feel slightly numb afterwards.

Vertical incisions

Midline

A midline incision is the most common general approach to the abdomen. It is used because the scar passes through the tissue joining the two large rectus muscles (the *linea alba*), and so no muscle tissue is actually cut. In the upper abdomen the scar extends from the middle of the lowest ribs (*xiphoid process*) to just above the tummy button (umbilicus). If more room is needed, the scar may be lengthened by taking it around and then below the umbilicus. With any operation what you see on the surface disguises the amount of tissue that has been cut. To get to an organ, the surgeon must cut through skin, the fat layer beneath, the muscle (or in this case linea alba) and finally the *peritoneum* or lining of the abdominal cavity which consists of sheets of connective tissue holding the organs in place.

Paramedian

A paramedian incision is parallel to the midline approach above, but about 3 cm from the midline. More tissue is cut through now, because the surgeon must cut into the covering layer of the rectus muscle, the *rectus sheath*. The rectus muscle fibres are divided rather than cut. The nerves and blood vessels on the outer (lateral) side of the muscle can be affected by a paramedian incision, so the muscle tends to appear wasted after surgery and take more time to build back up.

Transverse and oblique incisions

Subcostal

The subcostal or *kocher* incision is often used for gall bladder operations. As it is performed at the top end of the abdomen, less tissue is cut through, making it useful for an obese individual. With this incision, the rectus abdominis, internal oblique and transversus abdominis muscles are all cut and any small blood vessels that bleed will be *cauterised* (sealed with heat), so the muscles will take more time to recover. Often a small nerve (the eighth thoracic nerve) may be cut as well, delaying muscle recovery slightly.

McBurney

The McBurney incision is most commonly used for *appendix* operations. It is made about 2 cm above (proximal) to the sharp front edge of the pelvis (the anterior superior iliac spine) on the right side of the body. The incision runs parallel to the fibres of the external oblique muscle fibres, so these muscles are separated and retracted rather than cut, speeding post-surgical recovery.

Lower uterine (bikini)

The lower uterine incision is normally used with a caesarian section (c-section), and is made across the lower abdomen, just above the top of the bladder. Sometimes a midline (vertical) incision may be used if the baby is very large. C-sections are used in about 20 per cent of births in the UK. This procedure is normally carried out using regional anaesthesia – that is an *epidural* or spinal painkiller where the mother remains awake. Again, muscles are not cut, but the rectus muscles are separated and stretched. Recovery usually only takes about four days.

Hernia

A hernia occurs when tissue presses through a weakened area of the body, and hernias can occur in many body regions. For example, you can get a hernia on the back of the knee (Baker's cyst) where the knee joint capsule presses through the gap between the muscles at the back of the knee. However, most people think of the abdominal region when hernia is mentioned, and we will focus on this area. There are several types of hernia, the most common being the *inguinal* hernia.

Inguinal hernia

An inguinal or 'groin' hernia is the most common type of hernia in adults. It is seen more frequently in men and occurs due to weakness in the abdominal wall. The hernia presses through a naturally weak region in the lower abdomen called the *myopectineal orifice* (MPO). This small area has no strong muscle tissue reinforcing it. Above the MPO is an arch formed from fibres of the *internal oblique* and *transversus* muscle. Medially (towards the centre of the body) is the *rectus abdominis* muscle, with its covering sheath, and laterally (to the outside of the body) lies the *iliopsoas* muscle. At the bottom of the MPO is the pectineal ligament near the pubic region of the pelvis.

> ### Keypoint
>
> An inguinal hernia passes through a naturally weakened area between the lower abdominal muscles.

The inguinal hernia appears as a bulge just above the groin crease, close to the pubic area. The bulge is often made larger when coughing or sneezing, and when straining. In about 10 per cent of patients this type of hernia occurs on both sides of the body, which is known as a bilateral inguinal hernia.

An inguinal hernia can either be congenital (also called indirect) or acquired (also called direct). A congenital hernia is present from birth and occurs due to natural weakness in the muscles, and may be present for some years before it is noticed. An acquired hernia occurs as a result of repeated stress on the muscles through activities such as heavy lifting/straining, and excessive abdominal muscle training which causes the lower abdominal muscles to tear.

Pain from a hernia may appear as a dull ache in the groin and can travel (called referred pain) into the testicle and lower back. It may be intermittent and become quite severe at times only to disappear for hours at a time. Straining, muscle contraction and hip stretching movements will often make the pain worse.

Femoral hernia

In contrast to the inguinal hernia, a *femoral* hernia is more common in women. Again, it occurs in the groin area but this time slightly below the groin crease in a weak area called the femoral triangle. This triangle is formed between the groin crease (inguinal ligament) at the top, the long adductor muscles medially and the sartorius muscle laterally. The femoral triangle is slightly larger in women because of the wider pelvis compared to men, hence this hernia is more common in women.

Other hernias

Umbilical and incisional hernia

As the name suggests, an *umbilical* hernia occurs around the umbilicus or tummy button. It is associated with obesity where the abdominal wall is stretched, and the bulge can simply turn the normal inner contour of the umbilicus (an innie) into a dome (an outie). An incisional hernia occurs in a region of a previous operation scar – an important consideration when re-starting exercise following surgery.

Sports hernia

A sports hernia can give pain in the same region as an inguinal hernia, the difference being that there is no bulge on straining. A sports hernia is an inflammation of the lower abdominal muscles and attaching tissue (fascia) as they attach into the groin. Treatment can be surgical if the condition is severe and there is actual tissue damage. Frequently patients with this condition will recover with rest (anything up to six weeks) followed by correct strengthening and stretching of the abdominal muscles.

Hernia treatment

Herniae are usually found by a doctor or physiotherapist through a combination of history and examination. The history is normally one of strain to the lower abdomen. At examination, pain is in a characteristic location and normally increases with strain and muscle contraction. For a very minor hernia, ultrasound examination is often used. As the patient strains, a small bulge can be seen to pass through the tissue wall and move back when the strain is released. For general hernia a bulge will be seen on straining.

Hernia repair – what the surgeon does

Two types of operations are used when repairing a hernia. An open repair is usually done under a full anaesthetic and involves the surgeon making an 8 cm (3.2 inch) cut into the groin. The piece of tissue forming the hernia (*hernia sac*) is either pushed back inside the body or cut away. A plastic mesh is placed over the back of the weakened area that the hernia has passed through and is stitched into place. The skin covering the mesh is stitched together using dissolving stitches.

When using keyhole surgery, three small cuts of 0.5–1.5 cm (0.2–0.6 inches) are made into the lower abdomen. A balloon is passed through the largest hole and inflated to create a space in which the operation is performed. Gas is blown into the space to inflate it and the balloon is removed. Small instruments are inserted through tubes placed in the smaller incisions and the operation is conducted. A plastic mesh is stitched into place over the hernia area and the skin is stitched back together with dissolving stitches. As the keyholes are much smaller than the cut used in an open repair, skin healing is faster.

In both cases of hernia repair, the surgeon is careful to use a tension-free technique. Rather than simply stitching the two edges of the hernia defect (the hole through which the hernia passed), mesh is used. If the defect is simply stitched and pulled together, the stitches would cut into the tissue causing further tissue damage. The hernia defect is left as it is (the edges of the hole remaining relaxed) and the plastic mesh placed over it.

Abdominal exercise following surgery

Following surgery it is essential that abdominal muscle contraction is redeveloped. A combination of the original injury, pain which spreads throughout the area, and the altered muscle structure following surgery, means that it is often very difficult for individuals to get their abdominal muscles working correctly again. Let's take a look at a typical post-operation programme to aid recovery. Always remember, however, that your surgeon and physiotherapist have direct knowledge of your body and your condition so they may vary the programme according to your needs.

Immediate post-operative period

Immediately after your operation you have two concerns. The first is the effect of the anaesthetic on your body in general, the second is how to cope with daily living activities when your lower tummy is sore. At this stage don't try to do any abdominal exercises at all; just let your body recover – there will be time to exercise later. If you have had an open repair your scar will be larger and so even more sore. With a general anaesthetic you have inhaled gas into your lungs whereas with a local anaesthetic you are less likely to feel groggy. Make sure that you drink plenty of fluids as you may feel dry and dehydrated after your operation, and also eat some fruit. If you are dehydrated you may get constipated, and passing a dry stool will make you strain and may be very painful. Check the dressing which covers your scar – it will have dry fluid and blue-black dried blood on it. It you see any seepage from the dressing check back with your nurse or surgeon. Try to get out into the fresh air and perform some deep breathing exercises – breathe deeply, fill your lungs and breathe out completely. Perform 5 repetitions and then breathe normally for a minute. Repeat 3 times (15 reps in total with a 1 minute rest after each 5). This will help to flush any remaining anesthetic gases from your lungs and reduce post-operative fatigue.

When you move, your scar may pull slightly and hurt. This can be eased by supporting your scar with the flat of your hand or a large, soft pillow; press gently to ease the pain.

Keypoint

The day after an operation involving a general anaesthetic, perform deep breathing exercises to clear any remaining an anaesthetic gases from your lungs.

2–5 days after your operation

You will now have had two nights sleep and 48 hours for your tissues to begin healing. It will take 3–4 days for your body to begin to create a healing bridge of new tissue across your wound, and about 3 weeks for your scar to become fully strong. At this stage what you don't do is probably more important than what

you do. Make sure that although you support your scar, you don't bend over when you walk. Try to walk tall, perhaps having a 5–10 minute walk on the flat at a moderate pace. Don't lift anything and avoid straining when going to the toilet. Keep up the fluids and the high fibre diet with plenty of fruit and vegetables.

It is normal to notice some bruising coming out at this stage as blood released at the time of your surgery works it way to the surface. As gravity pulls blood downwards, you may notice the bruising below your scar and into your upper thigh and testicle. If your testicle begins to swell, have your surgeon check this out.

You can use an ice pack over your scar to ease swelling. Use a dry ice pack wrapped in a clean tea towel (take care not to get your dressing wet). Keep it on for 10–15 minutes and reapply every 2–3 hours throughout the waking day.

After 3 days it is time to begin tentative core stability work. Use pelvic floor contractions (exercises 84–86, pages 175–7) and abdominal hollowing in sitting (exercise 16, page 93) or standing (exercise 18, page 95) while leaning against a wall. Gently contract the lower abdominal muscles, drawing your tummy inwards without holding your breath. You may find it difficult at first to contract your lower abdominal muscles so a couple of physiotherapy 'tricks of the trade' may help. Firstly, use *tactile cueing*. Actually touch the part of the muscle that you want to contract. This will help to focus your brain onto this bodypart. Also, use *visualisation* – actually imagine that the muscle is contracting. Again this will draw the brain's attention into the muscle. When you do feel a gentle contraction beneath your fingers, *repeated contractions*, (physio techniques used on severely injured muscle) may help. Tighten your muscles, then relax them but don't allow them to relax completely. Before they do, contract them again trying to make the muscle firmer still. Again, after this repetition relax only partially and contract for a third and final repetition. This repeated contraction technique allows the muscle to ramp up its contraction; you will often achieve a stronger contraction than if you used three standard repetitions with a rest after each.

In this post-operative stage one of the complications is wound infection. One of the first signs is that you develop a temperature, so it is important to take your temperature after your operation if you feel unwell. See your GP immediately if you have a temperature as they can prescribe medication to tackle the infection before it gets worse.

6–14 days after your operation

After five to six days, your scar should be healing well and you are ready to increase the amount of exercise that you are doing. You should still avoid strenuous activity, including heavy lifting, pushing/pulling, and sit-ups/crunches in the gym. Faster walking and light jogging is OK, but you are not yet ready to progress to full running or sprinting. Gradually build up both your abdominal strength and your general fitness. Progress from abdominal hollowing actions (exercises 14–18, pages 91–5) to limb loading actions (exercises 23–29, pages 103–9). Use lunges and squats to build leg power in preparation for lifting and pushing motions.

Back to work

After 14 days you should be back to your normal activities, albeit at a slightly less intense level. You may not be able to train as long because you will have lost some of your trunk fitness. Your general CV fitness and whole body strength may have suffered due to the pain incurred with your original injury, and the subsequent prolonged rest. The key message now is *progression*, both of your general exercise programme and general daily activities. When you try an exercise or an activity in the home, if it is painful, stop, rest, and begin again at a less intense level. If that is not painful (it might be slightly sore but should not cause actual pain) keep doing the activity until you are confident with it. After a further 3–5 days try the original action again and you will normally find that you are able to do it pain free.

Take as an example, reaching up to clean a high window. As you stretch right up, you may feel the region of your scar pulling. Stop and rest until the pain subsides, and then re-start just reaching to chest level. Try using the window cleaning action at this height simply as an exercise. When it is less painful and you have loosened off the stiffness, reach up slightly further. Each time you reach higher you should feel your lower abdominal region stretching but not becoming painful. If we were to score pain on a scale of 1 to 10 with 1 being virtually no pain and 10 being the worst pain imaginable, as you stretch your should feel no more than a 3 or 4 on the pain scale.

Although we are being wisely cautious, you must not become over-protective. There is no reason why following a hernia operation you should not get back to full strenuous exercise. The key is to build up exercise and daily activity gradually, but also to make sure that you eventually take it to an intense level. I would expect you to have full functional use by 6–8 weeks after a minor abdominal operation such as a hernia; you will be able to lift, push, pull, run and train normally. If you cannot, make an appointment with a physiotherapist to have them guide you through an individualised programme.

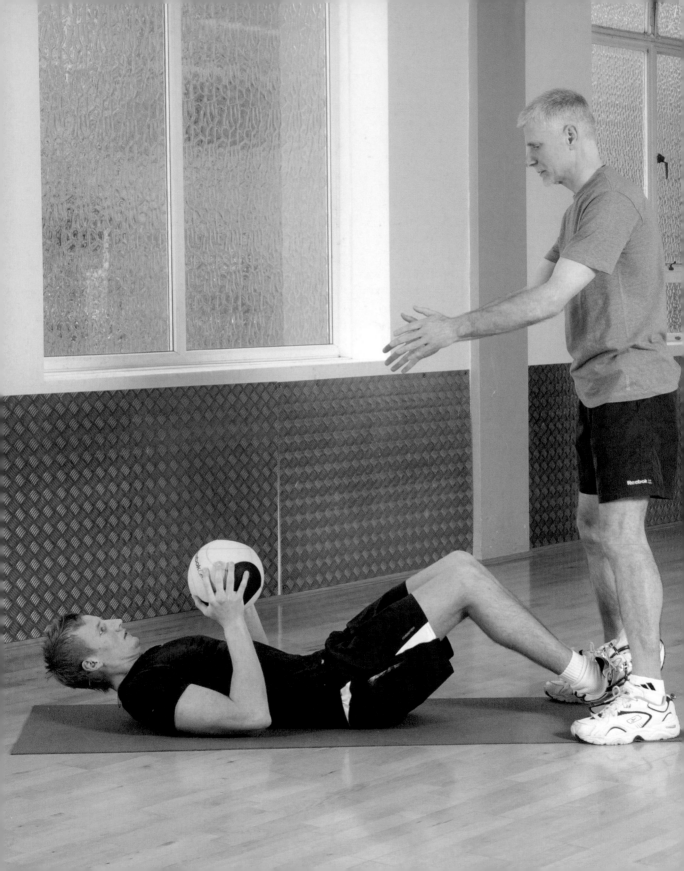

ABDOMINAL MUSCLE RESEARCH 17

The exercises used in this book are based on modern training methods developed for both cutting edge rehabilitation and high level sports training. These have gradually filtered down to the general public. Because discoveries are being made constantly, however, our knowledge must continually be updated. By looking at some of the research into abdominal training we can see at first hand how the developments begin and how they will affect our normal training programmes.

Effects of core stability on general abdominal training

We saw in chapter 2 that the core stability muscles (transversus and internal oblique especially) tighten and pull the abdominal wall flat, while the external oblique and rectus muscles actually move the trunk against resistance. But, if we practise core stability and perfect the abdominal hollowing technique (exercises 14–18, pages 91–5) how will this change the way we perform normal abdominal exercises in the gym such as sit-up, crunches, and leg raises? Part of the answer to this question was discussed in chapter 6 when we saw that abdominal doming is caused by performing an abdominal exercise without firstly hollowing the abdominal wall by working the core stabilisers. Researchers at

James Cook University in Australia[1] used EMG recording of the abdominal muscles to determine the difference between performing a standard abdominal exercise, and of performing the same exercise but using abdominal hollowing first. They found that by initiating the exercise with hollowing, subjects did indeed activate their transversus and internal obliques muscles before their rectus. This process is called *selective recruitment* and is an important method of dictating the order in which a group of muscles contracts. It confirms the importance of hollowing to 'set' the stability of the trunk before performing any sit-up type exercise.

Keypoint

Use the core muscles to 'set' the abdomen before all general abdominal exercise actions.

How effective are new abdominal exercises?

Exercises such as sit-ups and leg raises have been used since Victorian times, and crunches and trunk curls became fashionable in the late 1960s and early 1970s. The 1980s saw research into spinal stabilisation and the gradual adoption

---

[1] Barnett, F., and Gilleard, W. (2005), 'The use of spinal stabilisation techniques during the performance of abdominal strengthening exercise variations', *Journal of Sports Medicine and Physical Fitness,* 45(1), pp. 38–43

of these exercises into the fitness world under the general term 'core exercise'. Instructors and manufacturers are continually inventing new exercises and training devices in the search for better movements, but are these exercises really better, or just more of the same? This was the subject of research from California State University in Sacramento[2].

These researchers looked at three exercises: an abdominal frame (exercise 47, page 128); hanging knee raise (exercise 73, page 158) using straps; and a 'powerwheel' which is a commercial exercise similar to exercise 56, page 138. They found that the powerwheel gave the most intense muscle contraction and used the spinal muscles and latissimus dorsi as well, indicating its use as an overall stabilising movement. The powerwheel also activated the hip muscles due to the leg motion involved. These new exercises are effective for general stabilising movements, but not for muscle isolation actions.

Abdominal exercise dangers

Many physiotherapists and personal trainers stress the importance of correctly performed abdominal exercises, and in chapter 7 we saw some of the potential dangers of poor exercise technique. But does research support this approach?

One of the most important teaching points of sit-up type exercises is to warn users not to link their hands behind their neck and pull the head forwards (cervical flexion). Neurosurgeons in Denton, USA[3] described the tragic case of a 14-year-old boy who was a competitive wrestler. This subject performed sit-ups with his hands behind his head as part of a daily fitness routine. After one such workout he suddenly experienced total loss of movement (paresis) of his arms and weakness of his legs. He was rushed to hospital and underwent an MRI scan. One of the ligaments (ligamentum flavum) in his neck had been stretched so forcefully that it compressed his spinal cord, effectively cutting off its blood supply. This type of injury is normally only ever seen in older people who have severe degeneration of the bones in their neck. Thankfully the teenager recovered, but this case should sound a warning bell in every gym. Had this boy pulled a little bit harder or exercised slightly longer in this workout he may have been permanently paralysed.

Keypoint

To use your hands for neck support, place them lightly at the side of your head and do not pull the neck into flexion.

Doctors from the department of neurology at Penn State College of Medicine in America[4] again looked at sit-up exercises, but this time at the tragic effects of holding the breath (valsalva maneuver) while straining to perform the exercise. An important teaching point with resistance exercise is to keep breathing – 'breathe out on effort' is an old adage still familiar to most gym users. These two reports showed what happened when exercisers did not adhere to this practice.

[2] Escamilla, R.F., Babb, E., Dewitt, R. et al (2006), 'Electromyographic analysis of traditional and non-traditional abdominal exercises: Implications for rehabilitation and training', *Physical Therapy*, 86(5), pp. 656–71

[3] Dickerman, R.D., Mittler, M.A., Warshaw, C., and Epstein, J.A. (2005), 'Spinal cord injury in a 14-year-old male secondary to cervical hyperflexion with exercise', *Spinal Cord*, Aug 30

[4] Uber-Zak, L.D, and Venkatesh, Y.S. (2002), 'Neurologic complications of sit-ups associated with the Valsalva manoeuvre: Two case reports', *Archives of Physical Medicine and Rehabilitation*, 83(2), pp. 278–82

The first report was of a 37-year-old male who had been using rapid sit-ups without breathing correctly. He suddenly developed right-sided weakness and loss of sensation and was rushed to hospital. When there, it was noticed that his facial muscles on the right side had dropped and his strength reduced. In short, he had suffered a stroke! Over the next few days he developed a severe headache and a scan revealed that one of the most import-ant blood vessels going to his brain (posterior cerebral artery) had been blocked. After five days he began to improve, but required inten-sive neurological physiotherapy to recover.

The second case was a 30 year old who trained using 'hard, fast sit-ups' for a prolonged period without having time to breathe correctly. He developed neck pain, which travelled into his chest, and weakness of his arms and legs. An MRI scan showed that he had bled into the tube protecting his spinal cord (extradural haematoma). This blood had to be surgically removed and the subject required intense physiotherapy to recover. This type of injury would have required signifi-cant force to produce and would normally be seen after a car accident, for example.

These reports illustrate an important combin-ation of two actions: breath holding (Valsalva) and trunk flexion. Breath holding has been shown to change blood flow to the brain by compressing the major blood vessels which travel inside the trunk. Trunk flexion will also produce this effect by effectively crushing the body organs against the same deep blood vessels. When these two effects are combined, the blood pressure changes can have very serious effects.

> **Keypoint**
>
> Breathe normally throughout abdominal exercises. Do not hold your breath.

Which muscles work?

Researchers in Brazil[5] looked at 12 different abdominal exercises to distinguish between the work done by the abdominal muscles themselves, and that done by the hip flexor muscles – in particular the rectus femoris, which is the large 'kicking muscle' on the front of the thigh. They compared the upper and lower portions of the rectus abdominis muscle of the abdomen in 20 physical education students, and showed that, while leg lifting activities reduced the work on the upper rectus and emphasised the work on the lower portion of the muscle, bending the knees had little effect on the amount of work that the two portions of the muscle performed. Leg lift exercises produced the hardest workloads for the rectus femoris muscle, while curl-up actions produced the lightest. Fixing the feet increased the activity of the rectus femoris still further.

> **Keypoint**
>
> Sit-up type actions emphasise the upper portion of the rectus abdominis, while leg lift movements emphasise the lower portion. Fixing the feet will increase the work on the hip flexor muscles without any real advantage to the abdominal muscles.

Researchers in Australia[6] have looked closely at the difference between the deep stabilising muscles

---

[5] Guimaraes, A. C., Vaz, M. A., De Campos, M. I., Marantes, R. (1991), 'The contribution of the rectus abdominis and rectus femoris in 12 selected abdominal exercises: an electromyographic study', *Journal of Sports Medicine and Physical Fitness*, vol. 31:2, pp. 222–30

[6] O'Sullivan, P. B., Twomey, L. T., and Allison, G. T. (1997), 'Evaluation of specific stabilising exercise in the treatment of chronic low back pain with radiologic diagnosis of spondylolysis or spondylolisthesis', *Spine*, vol. 22:7, pp. 2959–67

(the transversus abdominis, multifidus and internal obliques) and the surface abdominal muscles (rectus abdominis and external obliques). When abdomal hollowing (*see* exercise 15) the internal oblique muscles work harder than the rectus abdominis muscle in most people. However, in people who have suffered long-standing lower back pain, the internal obliques work less and the rectus works more to try to compensate so that, as well as being weak, an imbalance is created between the two muscles (*see* fig. 17.1). In order to correct this imbalance, therefore, we must increase the work of the internal oblique muscles, and reduce the work of the rectus. Strengthening both

muscles will leave them stronger, but still out of balance.

It is also vital to distinguish between the deep muscles and those on the surface during training. The same researchers[7] looked at a 10-week programme using 15 minutes of core stability exercises (especially abdominal hollowing) daily, and compared this to a gym-based programme involving trunk curls and weights. Over the training programme, those using core stability exercises showed a dramatic increase in the activity of the internal oblique muscles but little change in the rectus. Those on the gym-based programme, however,

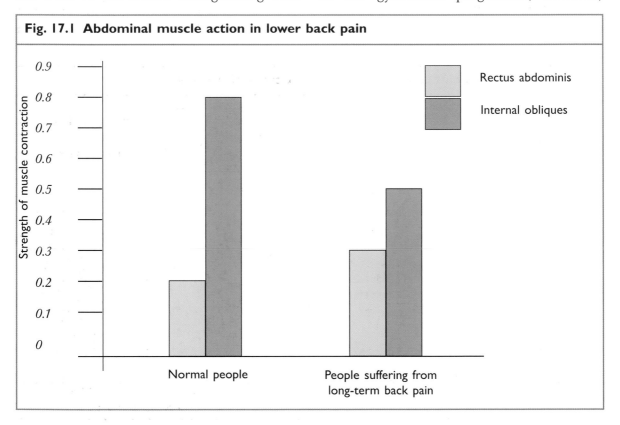

Fig. 17.1 Abdominal muscle action in lower back pain

Strength of muscle contraction — Normal people; People suffering from long-term back pain. Legend: Rectus abdominis; Internal obliques.

[7] O'Sullivan, P. B., Twomey, L. T., and Allison, G. T. (1998), 'Altered abdominal recruitment in patients with chronic back pain following a specific exercise intervention', *Journal of Orthopedic and Sports Physical Therapy*, vol. 27, pp. 114–24

showed an improvement in both rectus and internal oblique activity. Although in this case the muscles were stronger after the more traditional gym-based programme, the imbalance between the two sets of muscles still remained (*see* fig. 17.2).

Keypoint

A muscle imbalance exists in people with back pain whereby the stabilising muscles are not used enough and the surface abdominal muscles are used too much. To correct this imbalance, core stability exercises rather than normal gym-based programmes are required initially.

Physiotherapists at King's College, London[8], looked at the best method to work the transversus muscle (*see* fig. 2.1). They took 20 people and, using the kneeling position, gave half abdominal hollowing on its own, and the other half abdominal hollowing with pelvic-floor contraction. After six weeks the physios then looked at the thickness of the transversus muscle using ultrasound scanning. Abdominal hollowing by itself increased the thickness of the transversus by 49.7 per cent while abdominal hollowing with additional pelvic-floor contraction increased the muscle thickness by 65.8 per cent, a significantly higher score.

This study clearly shows the importance of linking the hollowing action to its normal

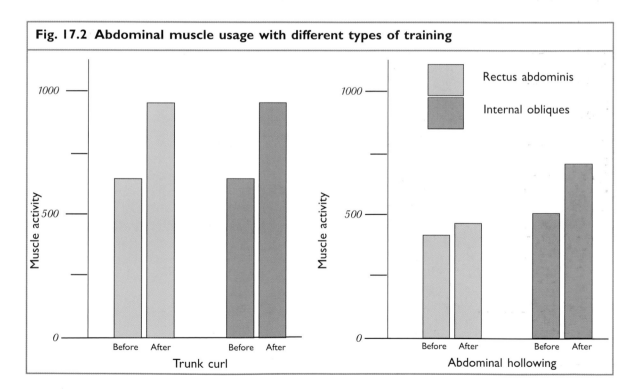

Fig. 17.2 Abdominal muscle usage with different types of training

Rectus abdominis

Internal obliques

Muscle activity — Trunk curl (Before, After, Before, After)

Muscle activity — Abdominal hollowing (Before, After, Before, After)

---

[8] Critchley, D. J. (2000), 'Instructing pelvic floor contraction increases transversus abdominis activation in low abdominal hollowing', Proceedings of the Chartered Society of Physiotherapy Congress (Birmingham, UK) p. 22

function in the body. We have seen that hollowing works as part of the abdominal balloon mechanism (*see* chapter 1) whereby the abdomen can be viewed as a cylinder with the deep stabilising muscles being the walls and the pelvic-floor muscles the base. Working both muscles at the same time is more effective than simply working one muscle in isolation because the body already recognises the coordination of the muscles pulling together to increase the pressure within the abdominal balloon.

> ### Keypoint
>
> Working the pelvic floor muscles with the deep stabilising muscles is an effective method to re-learn core stability.

Stress on the spine

When performing a sit-up-type activity, poorly trained people often allow the lower spine (lumbar region) to hollow excessively, a posture that greatly stresses the spine. This increased lumbar hollow, or 'lordosis', occurs because the abdominal muscles may be too weak to stabilise the spine or the person may simply not be using the muscles correctly. Researchers in Japan[9] looked at the effect of both muscle tensing, and head and neck position, when performing abdominal exercises. They found that sit-up type actions which involved bending (flexing) the neck and drawing the chin in towards the chest combined with abdominal stabilisation

through 'pulling the abdomen in', produced the best results in terms of muscle work. They also X-rayed the spine and showed that pulling the chin in and tightening (stabilising) the abdomen produced the least hollow back and therefore the safest exercise for the lumbar spine.

Researchers at the University of Iowa in America looked at curl exercises and a leg lowering task to determine the effect that a posterior pelvic tilt (pulling the abdomen tight and flattening the back) would have on the abdominal muscles[10]. They used EMG to look at the electrical activity of the rectus abdominis, and internal and external oblique muscles in 15 people while they performed either a trunk curl or double straight leg lowering exercise. When people performed the exercises in a neutral position, the rectus abdominis muscle and external obliques dominated the action with little work on the internal obliques. However, when a posterior pelvic tilt was maintained throughout the action, the activity of the rectus was reduced and that of the external and internal obliques significantly increased.

> ### Keypoint
>
> Drawing the tummy in (stabilising) and tucking the chin in when performing abdominal exercises helps to prevent the spine from curving inwards excessively and acts to protect it. To prevent excessive curvature in the lower back, posteriorly tilt the pelvis (flatten your back).

[9] Shirado, O., Ito, T., Kaneda, K. and Strax, T. E. (1995), 'Electromyographic analysis of four techniques for isometric trunk muscle exercises', *Archives of Physical Medicine and Rehabilitation*, vol. 76:3, pp. 225–9

[10] Shields, R. K., Heiss, D. G. (1997), 'An electromyographic comparison of abdominal muscle synergies during curl and double straight leg lowering exercises with control of the pelvic position', *Spine*, vol. 22:16, pp. 1873–9

Researchers from Sweden[11] looked at the effect of abdominal training on intra-abdominal pressure in both healthy people and those with a history of lower back pain. They gave each a series of bent knee curl-ups to do while holding their breath – 2 sets of 10 curl-ups daily over 5 weeks, during which time both the holding time and resistance of the exercise were gradually increased. The strength of the abdominal muscles increased but the intra-abdominal pressure did not. The authors concluded that the people could not make functional use of their increased strength because the pattern of movement in training was different from that during lifting.

Scientists from the Department of Neuroscience at the Karolinska Institute in Stockholm, Sweden[12] looked at the effect of a 10-week specific abdominal strength programme which targeted resisted trunk rotations. Rotation strength increased by nearly 30 per cent after training, and the rate of intra-abdominal pressure development during jumping activities and trunk pushing actions also increased. They therefore concluded that an increase in strength of the trunk rotator muscles with training also increased the rate of intra-abdominal pressure development during functional – in other words, real-life – situations.

> ## Keypoint
>
> To increase the power of the 'abdominal balloon', the deep stabilising muscles must be used. Exercises which fail to train these muscles may increase strength and fitness, but will not significantly improve core stability.

Abdominal training and appearance

Individuals often begin a gym programme with the sole intension of flattening the tummy or 'toning and trimming' the waist. Many researchers have looked at the ability of abdominal training to alter appearance in this way and their findings can be used to guide us to better exercise programmes.

Researchers at the University of Massachusetts[13] looked at the effect of sit-up exercises on the amount of fat around the waist. To assess 'fatness', they used body girth measurements using a tape measure, skin folds measurements and total fat content using a special machine to detect the amount of fatty tissue in the body. Initially the people in this study undertook an average of 140 sit-ups each day in the first week, and increased this to

[11] Hemborg, B., Moritz, S. and Hamberg, J. (1985), 'Intra-abdominal pressure and trunk muscle activity during lifting – effect of abdominal muscle training in chronic low back patients', *Scandinavian Journal of Rehabilitation Medicine*, vol. 17, pp. 15–24

[12] Cresswell, A. G., Blake, P. L., and Thorstensson, A. (1994), 'The effect of an abdominal muscle training programme on intra-abdominal pressure', *Scandinavian Journal of Rehabilitation Medicine*, vol. 26:2, pp. 79–86

[13] Katch, F. I. (1984), 'Effects of sit-up exercise training on adipose cell size and adiposity', *Research Quarterly for Exercise and Sports*, vol. 55, p. 242

336 sit-ups per day by the end of the 27-day training period. The scientists found that there was no real change in any of the fatness measures by the end of the programme. The people were certainly stronger and able to perform a greater number of sit-ups, so muscle training had definitely taken place. However, this training did not include a reduction in body fatness, because this type of training tones and strengthens the muscles. To reduce body fat we need a combination of diet and aerobic (fat burning) exercise such as cycling, jogging or swimming because it increases the 'tick over' of the body (measured as heart rate) for a prolonged period and burns energy in the form of Calories and ultimately fat.

Maintaining the theme of body appearance, at the University of Norfolk in the US, physical therapy researchers looked at the relationships between lumbar lordosis (low back hollow), pelvic tilt and abdominal muscle performance[14]. We know that lax abdominal muscles can lead to an increased lordosis, and is commonly seen, for example, in obesity and after pregnancy (*see* pages 42–4). However, is there a link between muscle strength and this type of posture? In other words, if your abdominal muscles are stronger, do you have a better posture?

These researchers took 31 physical therapy students and measured their lumbar lordosis and pelvic tilt angle. They then assessed the strength of the abdominal muscles, emphasising the lower (infra-umbilical) part of the rectus abdominis muscle by using a leg lowering task. The students lay on a gym bench, holding on to it above their heads for stability, and were then helped to lift their legs to a vertical pos-

ition. They then lowered their legs on their own taking 10 seconds to do so, being instructed to keep their backs flat against the bench. As soon as their back began to lift from the bench, the exercise was stopped and the leg angle at which this happened was noted.

The researchers found that there was no relationship between abdominal muscle performance and pelvic tilt or lordosis. Why? The answer is that the abdominal muscles are largely relaxed in normal standing, only becoming active if the trunk is moved. In relaxed standing, it is the length of the abdominal muscles rather than their strength which is important, and when we stand in this fashion the muscles support us, not by contracting, but simply through elasticity. With obesity, over a period of time, the muscles sag and become overstretched, and it is this lengthening which is important from the point of view of relaxed posture.

Two physiotherapists from the University of Queensland in Australia[15] took up this idea and looked at the length of the muscles around the abdomen and the relationship with pelvic angle (pelvic tilt). They looked at 103 adolescent women using a specially designed pelvic angulation measuring device and found that the lengths of the abdominal muscles, the hamstrings and the erector spinae were highly related to lumbar lordosis and could actually be used to predict the depth of the lordosis likely to be found in a given person. This is precisely what is described in chapter 4, where the balance between the pull of the muscles around the pelvis is discussed. To change posture with exercise, it seems likely that a

[14] Walker, M. L., Rothstein, J. M., Finvcane, S. O. and Lamb, R. L. (1987), 'Relationships between lumbar lordosis, pelvic tilt and abdominal muscle performance', *Physical Therapy*, vol. 67:4, pp. 512–16

[15] Toppenberg, R. M., and Bullock, M. I. (1986), 'The interrelation of spinal curves, pelvic tilt and muscle lengths in the adolescent female', *Australian Journal of Physiotherapy*, vol. 32:1, pp. 6–12

combination of diet/weight loss with muscle balancing exercise is needed. To change pelvic tilt in obesity, we must reduce body fat, stretch the shortened hamstring muscles and shorten the lengthened abdominal muscles. This is achieved by a combination of deep muscle corset exercise together with the modified trunk curl movement (exercise 36, page 117).

Keypoint

To reduce your waistline you need a combination of diet and regular aerobic exercise. To change your posture you need muscle balancing, rather than pure strength training.

Fig. 17.3 Following the exercises in this book will help you towards the correct abdominal balance.

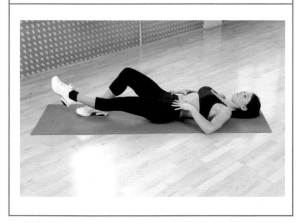

PLANNING YOUR ABDOMINAL TRAINING PROGRAMME 18

We have seen a great many exercises in this book. All are designed in some way to improve core stability, develop the condition of your abdominal muscles, and enhance the function of your trunk area. Some are basic, some more advanced. Many are used in combination with stretching or strength training, for example, to achieve core stability as part of an overall training plan. Some are worked in conjunction with postural correction. How do we put it all together to form a coherent abdominal training programme?

Your current abdominal muscle condition

Before we start to plan an abdominal training programme we must determine the current state of your abdominal muscles. To do this, we use four basic exercises as simple tests. These are designed to show not how good or bad your muscles are in terms of tone or strength, but to give you a point at which to start – *your baseline abdominal condition.*

The first exercise is abdominal hollowing, as used in exercise 18 (page 95) but with some modifications. It measures your ability firstly to perform an important muscle isolation, and secondly to hold the position – a test of muscle endurance.

Ex 99 Abdominal hollowing test

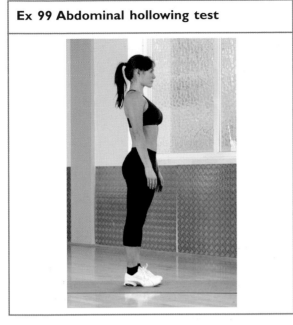

Starting position

Stand with your back flat against a wall and your feet forwards of the wall by 20 cm. You can place your thumbs inside the waistband of your trousers/shorts so that there is a small (1 cm) gap between your abdominal wall and the waistband.

Action

Focus your attention on your lower abdominal region. Breathe in and, as you breathe out, try to draw your abdominal wall away from your waistband. Hold this position for 10 seconds while breathing in and out normally.

Points to note

It is possible to get a false result on this test by drawing your abdominal wall in through simply taking a very big breath and lifting your ribcage. Make sure you breathe normally and keep your ribcage still through the exercise.

Training tip

If you find you are unable to hold the hollow position for 10 seconds, use the test as an exercise. Initially focus on holding for 1–2 seconds and build up the holding time. When you can hold for 10 seconds you have passed the test.

The next test measures your ability to use your core stabilising muscles to maintain the position of your spine as you move another part of your body. This is a vital function of the abdominals – to protect the spine and keep the correct alignment against forces acting on it. It is a modification of exercise 23.

Ex 100 Heel slide maintaining neutral position

(a)

(b)

(c)

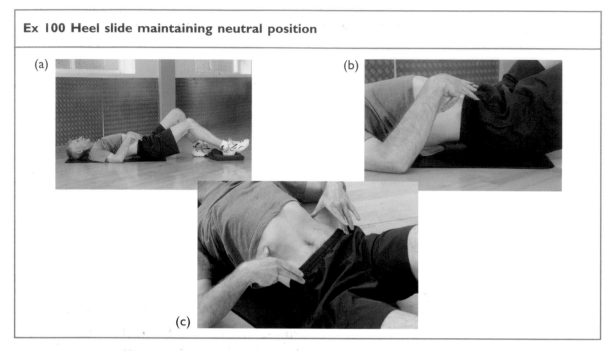

Starting position

Begin lying on the floor on a mat, with your knees bent and feet flat. Place your fingers lightly on the bones at the front of your pelvis (anterior superior iliac spines).

Action

Straighten your right leg, sliding the heel out over the floor. At the same time, use your fingers to monitor pelvic movement. The aim of the test is for you to be able to straighten firstly your right leg and then the left, without the pelvis moving.

Points to note

If you are very unstable in the lumbar spine, the pelvic movement is obvious. Your pelvis will tip forwards and the pelvic bones beneath your fingers will move downwards. As this happens your spine will hollow, increasing the gap between your back and the mat (b).

Training tip

If you are unable to hold the spine still, the test is failed. Practise exercise 15 (page 92) for 2–3 days until you are able to master the movement. Then use exercise 23 (page 103) and finally exercise 28 (page 108) until you are able to pass the test.

Ex 101 Single straight leg raise monitoring abdominal wall – (c) is incorrect

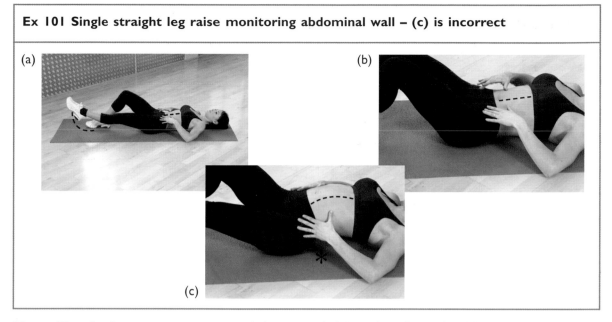

(a)

(b)

(c)

Note: The third test measures your ability to tighten your abdominal muscles and draw them in flat. We saw in chapter 2 that the transversus abdominis muscle draws the abdominal wall in while the rectus abdominis and external oblique move the spine and produce powerful actions. In chapter 17 research was highlighted which showed that the deep stabilisers should contract slightly before the superficial muscles to 'set' the abdomen before any movement occurs. This test is a measure of the setting function, using a modification of exercise 29 (page 109).

Starting position

Begin lying on the floor on a mat, with your legs straight. Spread your fingertips and place them about 1 cm above your abdomen.

Action

Raise and lower your right leg and then your left three times, each by 15–20 cm (a). At the same time pay attention to the contour of your abdominal wall; it should stay flat, so that it remains below your fingertips (b). If your abdominal wall bulges so that it touches your fingers, you have failed the test (c).

Points to note

This movement can be very subtle. If you find it difficult to monitor your abdominal wall, work with a partner. They can simply watch your abdomen to see if it bulges (fail) or stays flat (pass) as you lift your legs.

Training tip

If you fail this test, it means you have either weak core stabilisers, or a muscle imbalance where you surface abdominals are stronger than your deep stabilisers, particularly the transversus muscle. Practise exercise 15 (page 92) for 2–3 days until you are able to master the movement. Then use exercise 23 (page 103) for 2–3 days before re-testing yourself.

Ex 102 Straight leg sit-up, keeping legs down – (d) is incorrect

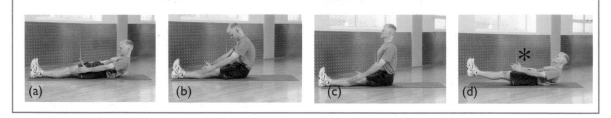

(a)   (b)   (c)   (d)

Note: The fourth test should only be attempted if you have passed tests 1–3, and if you have no history of back injury. It is a measure of both abdominal muscle strength, and your ability to shorten you rectus abdominis muscle enough to bend (flex) your spine to curl up rather than sit up straight. It is a monitored version of exercise 63 (page 145).

Starting position

Begin lying on the floor on a mat, with your legs straight and arms by your sides.

Action

Firstly bend your neck (drawing your chin inwards) to look at your feet (a). Tighten your abdominal muscles and flatten your back onto the mat and then curl (bend) your trunk (b) to sit up (c). Stop the exercise immediately if your legs begin to lift from the mat; when they lift, you have failed the test (d).

Points to note

This is a hard test for highly trained athletes who want to measure their abdominal performance. It must be performed slowly and stopped immediately if the legs lift. To continue the movement with the legs lifting or to perform the exercise quickly places an excessive stress on the lumbar spine. Some individuals naturally find this exercise difficult if they are heavy in the upper body and have lighter legs. Their body proportions are such that they cannot easily reduce the leverage action of the trunk sufficiently to perform the exercise correctly.

Training tip

If you are unable to sit up without your legs lifting, your abdominal muscles are usually lengthened. Perform exercise 36 (page 66) to shorten them.

Once you have the result of these tests you will have an idea of condition of the abdominal muscles and where to begin. If you were unable to hold the abdominal hollowing position in exercise 99, begin with this exercise and the other foundation movements. If you can hold the abdominal hollowing isolation movement, but cannot hold the neutral position during exercise 100, start with the level one exercises. For those who can perform the straight leg raise (exercise 101) without an abdominal bulge, begin with the more advanced movement of level one (exercise 29). If you tried exercise 101 but were unable to prevent your abdomen from bulging, then begin with the foundation movements focussing on abdominal hollowing. If you are an advanced athlete and were able to perform a straight leg sit-up without your legs lifting (exercise 102) you are ready for all of the level 3 exercises and capable of progressing to abdominal training with weights, and using power and speed movements.

Before you start

Before embarking on any exercise programme, you must warm up. Even if you are an advanced user, it is sensible to begin a training session with some of the foundation movements as this will 'rehearse' the skills of stability. The key skill is to be able to hollow the abdomen gently, and to maintain this muscle contraction over a period of time. This simple action will enable you to maintain alignment and the 'neutral position' of the lumbar spine (*see* exercise 10, page 86) throughout the exercise programme. Three to five repetitions is required, holding each for 10 seconds while breathing normally.

Let's now look at some examples of real-life ('functional') situations through some case studies. Remember that these are *examples* and may not exactly match your own requirements.

> ### Keypoint
>
> Rehearse abdominal hollowing before you start abdominal training, and aim to maintain the neutral position of the lumbar spine as often as you can during your workout.

If you have had an injury to the spine you should see a physiotherapist before embarking on core stability training. If you are unsure of your alignment or how to progress your exercise programme, work with a certified personal trainer or exercise professional.

The overweight individual

George is a 38 year old who is about 10 kg (22 lb) overweight. His body fat is 22 per cent and his waist measurement equals his age. A poor diet, too many business lunches and too much alcohol have all taken their toll. He looks and feels 50 and wants to do something about it, but does not know how.

Firstly, diet was the keystone of this programme. He needed to improve the *quality* of his food intake. Less alcohol combined with a reduction in sweet and fatty snack foods started to make an impression. Increasing his intake of fresh fruit and vegetables not only allowed him to lose body fat, but probably dramatically improved his health as well. His diet was combined with regular exercise, and he began with a 10-minute brisk walk each evening and one 20-minute swim each week. This will have increased his metabolic rate (body 'tick-over') for long periods after exercise had finished, and helped to burn calories as well as improve the health of his heart, lungs and circulation. In the first month his weight came down by 4 kg (9 lb) and his waistline reduced by 2.5 cm (1 inch).

George focused on a single abdominal exercise, performing abdominal hollowing standing with his back towards a wall (exercise 7, page 94). Initially he stood looking in a mirror, and also touched his abdominal wall with his fingertips to really appreciate what was happening (tactile cueing). By pulling his abdomen away from his waistband and holding the movement while breathing normally, he was able to build up the holding time.

He found the movement very hard to start with. Nothing seemed to happen, but eventually he was able to pull his abdomen from his waistband for 1 or 2 seconds and get the feeling of the exercise. After his first week, practising this movement three times a day, he was able to hold the exercise for 5 seconds. He still found it difficult to keep his ribcage still, but the skill was coming. By week three, George could hold the movement for over 5 seconds and put much less effort into the exercise. He could perform the action without touching his abdomen or looking in a mirror and now used the hollowing action when standing (while shaving in the morning) and also when walking. He found it easier to pull his abdomen away from his waistband for 10 steps and then to relax for 10 steps while out on his daily 10-minute walk.

After his first month George was ready to move on and began abdominal hollowing lying (exercise 15, page 92). From this position he moved on to the heel slide (exercise 23, page 103). Initially he started with three repetitions on each leg and built up to five and then eight. His diet was going well and his general exercise was increasing. He went to a local gym and began treadmill walking on the flat and then uphill. When his business commitments prevented him from visiting the gym he extended both the length of his walk (15 minutes) and its intensity (slow to begin, followed by 5 minutes' fast walking and slow to end). In addition, George used a cross-training machine in the gym (5 minutes) and the rowing machine (5 minutes). To finish off he performed some supervised lightweight training on the seated shoulder press and lateral pull down machine.

Programme
• Diet to reduce body fat • Cardiopulmonary exercise • Abdominal hollowing, standing (using belt) • Abdominal hollowing while walking • Heel slide

The individual with back pain
Julie had lower back pain after the birth of her second child. She was 28 and not overweight, although her body tone was less than it was when she was at college. Her children were aged four and six, and she had back pain especially when bending over to pick up her four year old. The pain was worse when she sat for a long time. It was often so bad that she found it hard to get to sleep as she could not easily lie flat.

It turned out Julie had a flatback posture, meaning that the normal curve in her lower back had become flattened out. Her abdominal muscles had poor tone and she had a little 'pot belly' below her umbilicus and, although her general flexibility was quite good, her hamstrings were unusually tight.

Initially Julie was given abdominal hollowing in kneeling position (exercise 14, page 91) as this was a position in which she had no back pain. She found it difficult to perform the exercise at first – she said that nothing seemed to happen in the tummy! The exercise programme was therefore amended so that it began with pelvic floor contractions (exercise 21, page 100). In conversation Julie admitted that she had not practised these after the birth of her second child and occasionally she 'dribbled' a little urine when she laughed or coughed. When the pelvic floor contractions were performed, Julie was encouraged to continue the feeling into her lower tummy and feel the umbilicus pulled inwards and upwards. She found this easier when a loose belt was placed around her waist as she was able to feel the muscles pulling away from something. Julie built up the abdominal hollowing to 10 repetitions, holding each for 3 seconds and eventually for 10 seconds, and she practised this twice daily.

To correct her flatback posture Julie did five low back extension stretches (exercise 8, page 52) three times a day. She found this movement quite stiff and sore to begin with but, as she persevered, the pain gradually eased and the back stretched loose. In addition, Julie was encouraged to practise good back care, limiting the amount of bending that she did and trying whenever possible to bend her knees.

When Julie could perform the abdominal hollowing action easily in the kneeling position (exercise 14, page 91), she began to practise the same movement both lying (exercise 15, page 92) and sitting (exercise 16, page 93), in each case performing 10 repetitions once a day. This led on to leg lowering from supine lying (exercise 29, page 109) and finally leg lowering from a crunch position (exercise 49, page 131). By this time Julie had joined an exercise class and so practised the abdominal training movements three times a week at home. Before each class, however, she still rehearsed abdominal hollowing, and was conscious of her alignment throughout the workout.

To stretch her tight hamstrings, Julie performed abdominal hollowing and leg straightening (exercise 28, page 108) occasionally during normal activities throughout the day.

Programme

• Pelvic-floor contractions • Abdominal hollowing, kneeling • Spinal extension stretch • Good back care during the day • Abdominal hollowing, lying and sitting • Leg lowering from supine lying • Leg lowering from crunch position • Abdominal hollowing and leg straightening

Poor stability in an athlete

Pooja was a regular at the local gym. She exercised daily, three times per week in the weights room and three aerobic classes, including step and jazz dance. Even at weekends she was active, mountain biking or going for a run. Examination of her trunk showed a classic 'six pack' and a lean, honed physique. However, she complained of lower back pain during, and especially the morning after, her weights programme. Two exercises gave her particular problems, the standing hip extension on a 'multi-hip' unit and repeated overhead pressing actions with a light aerobics bar. She reported soreness in the lower back developing gradually and building in intensity until she had to stop the exercise. On close examination of these movements it became obvious that she hyperextended her spine as she performed both actions. This meant that her pelvis tilted forwards (front part down) and her lower back arched forwards excessively. This is the classic lordotic posture, and on stretch tests her hip flexor muscles proved tighter than you would expect for a well-trained athlete.

Pooja's problem was not lack of strength, far from it – it was *imbalance*. For her physique and strength, she had very little proportional core stability. As she performed the exercises, her 'corset' muscles (deep abdominals) were unable to hold her spine firmly in its neutral position, and her tight hip flexor muscles were constantly pulling the front of her pelvis down. Her core stability was tested by giving her a heel slide exercise while lying on her back (exercise 100, page 214). After only four slow repetitions, her back began to arch away from the ground, whereas an athlete of her calibre should be able to perform 20–30 repetitions of this movement easily.

Pooja's training programme was modified and all exercises removed which tended to push the spine out of alignment. This included all overhead pressing actions and any hip extension movement. She spent the time saved by deleting these exercises on core stability training. The aim was to enhance core stability but, in addition (and in many ways more importantly), to improve her appreciation of alignment as well by being able to recognise when her spine began to move away from its neutral position. She began with abdominal hollowing in sitting (exercise 16, page 93) and standing positions (exercise 18, page 95) and was able to learn these actions quickly as her body awareness was excellent from the amount of time she had been exercising. She quickly moved up to leg lowering from a crunch position (exercise 38, page 119) and then progressed to the side lying body lift (exercise 46, page 127) and the spinal extension hold (exercise 72, page 157). In each case the precision of the movement was emphasised and Pooja was encouraged to perform the actions slowly, building up holding time (muscle endurance) to 30–45 seconds.

To retrain her neutral position recognition, Pooja performed pelvic tilting in lying (exercise 10, page 86), standing (exercise 11, page 87) and sitting positions (exercise 12, page 88). In each case she was required to move back into the neutral position without looking in the mirror, and with her eyes closed. This type of activity develops 'joint sense' – that is, the ability to recognise the position of a body part by feeling the movement rather than looking at it. This would be important in Pooja's general workout where she would be focusing on the moving weight rather than her mid-body. Pooja also began practising the kneeling hip flexor stretch (exercise 1, page 43), performing the movement slowly and maintaining her neutral spine position throughout the movement.

Finally, Pooja performed her normal gym workout with minimal weight resistance, focusing instead on alignment and maintaining the neutral position with her newly developed core stability. Only when she was able to do this was she allowed to increase her weights or the speed at which she practised her gym programme.

Programme

• Modified gym programme to remove stressful exercises • Abdominal hollowing, standing and sitting • Leg lowering from a crunch position • Side lying body lift • Spinal extension hold • Pelvic tilting activities • Hip flexor stretching • Alignment recognition and practice

INDEX OF EXERCISES

INDEX

NOTES

OTHER BOOKS BY CHRISTOPHER M. NORRIS

The Complete Guide to Stretching (3rd edn) (2007)

A reasonable level of flexibility is essential to the healthy functioning of joints and muscles, which in turn facilitates performance and reduces the risk of injury. This book provides an accessible overview of the scientific principles that underpin this form of training and offers more than 70 exercises designed to safely increase range of motion right across the body. This new edition is in full colour, with brand new photographs demonstrating the stretches throughout.

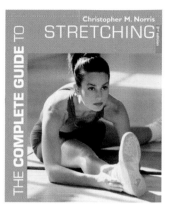

Bodytoning (2003)

More and more people are turning to weight training as a form of healthy exercise. In this book, renowned physiotherapist and author Chris Norris explains the principles behind weight training, including preparation, energy systems, how muscles work, and basic physiology, before taking the reader through a series of exercises, adaptable to all levels of ability. The emphasis is on safety throughout. Includes clear and comprehensive photographs and illustrations.

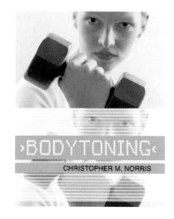

Available from all good bookshops or online. For more details on these and other A&C Black sport and fitness titles, please go to www.acblack.com.

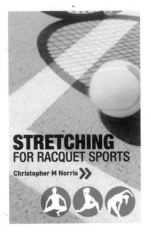

Stretching for Racquet Sports (2008)

Based on the hugely successful *Complete Guide to Stretching*, this new series is a sport-specific three-phase programme of stretching, from beginner level, through intermediate stretches, to advanced dynamic development. Small enough to keep in your sports bag, it includes advice on self-assessment and warm-ups, a training log to assess development, a section on treating injuries encountered in racquet sports and stretches illustrated with full-colour photographs.

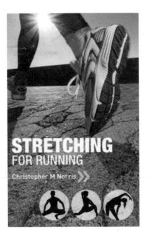

Stretching for Running (2008)

Part of the new **Stretching for...** series as outlined above, this title focuses on a three-phase programme of stretching, from beginner level, through intermediate stretches, to advanced dynamic development for running. Includes all of the same great features as *Stretching for Racquet Sports.*

Available from all good bookshops or online. For more details on these and other A&C Black sport and fitness titles, please go to www.acblack.com.